Social Stranger

Travis E. Breeding

ISBN: 1723526304
ISBN-13: 978-1723526305

DEDICATION

I would like to dedicate this to my friends and family. I also want to dedicate this to anyone who wants to learn more about autism and how it can effect some of us.

CONTENTS

Acknowledgments i

1   Coloring Outside the Lines   1

2   Distractions and Difficulties   5

3   The Last Kid Picked   16

4   Just Passing Through   25

5   Failing Socializing   34

6   Escape Into Fantasyland   48

7   Following Freshman   61

8   On the Outside Looking In   78

9   A Dream Discovered   96

10   A Chapter Closes   113

11   A Dream Dashed   173

12   Big Mistakes   208

13   Buying Love   241

14   Try Again   271

15   The Rebound   305

16   Lost   320

17   Reaching Out   334

About the Author   350

Di

ACKNOWLEDGMENTS

I would like to thank my friends and family
for being there for me and helping me
through my journey with autism.

1 COLORING OUTSIDE THE LINES

The preschool years were full of excitement and nervousness. I had never really had a friend before preschool as I grew up with two cousins very close in age and living nearby. What I remember most about preschool was swimming and trying to learn to play with the others. For some reason this wasn't very natural for me. Now that I know of my diagnoses it makes perfectly good sense. I did manage to make an acquaintance with another kid by the name of Eric. We kind of got to know who each other were I guess you could say. I can't remember a whole lot of the preschool years, but I think it's safe to say that Eric and I probably played together some at that level.

I remember some of the activities we were doing in preschool involving learning how to color and other's that included anything from cutting things out to gluing them to paper. All these activities are something that should be easy for any child to learn how to do. However, for me it was different for some reason and I'd always wondered why. I could never stay in the lines and it always hurt my hand and fingers when I had to color for an extended period. Cutting wasn't much easier for me as I struggled in just knowing and understanding how to hold the scissors. To me coloring, cutting, and gluing seemed so uninteresting and pointless. Maybe it was because it was very hard for me to do.

Meanwhile after the preschool years came time to go to Kindergarten. At five years old here I was ready to go off to school for the next thirteen years of my life. I think I had mixed emotions about this. In the fall of 1990 I went to Kindergarten round-up at Andrews Elementary School. My parents were there with me and I remember that the teacher had all kinds of activities for the children to do. She also talked a little about school. It did seem quite overwhelming to me.

As a kid I had many difficulties with fine motor skills. For example, I would often just randomly have a tick and shake my head and have no control over it. In fact, to this day this is still an issue for me except for now that I'm constantly aware of the possibility of it randomly happening I'm better able to prevent it. I also had problems with other fine motor skills such as balancing or standing on one foot. Throwing and catching. I would say that hand eye coordination was a huge problem for me. Even little things such as holding a pencil or crayon properly were a huge issue. So, after the Kindergarten round-up my parents and the teacher conferred and decided that it was best for me to wait and start Kindergarten a year later. This meant that I would not start Kindergarten until I was six. To this day I am not sure how I feel about that. I mean, I'm sure there were many pros to having that extra year to try and develop my skill set but at the same time it made me a year older than most of the other kids as I started Kindergarten in the fall of 1991. Here I was a six-year-old sitting in a classroom with a bunch of five-year old's.

Then the experience began. In late August of 1991 I started Kindergarten. Luckily for me I would have a great teacher. Mrs. Price was very understanding and caring. I remember having to use the bathroom a lot. Probably more so than most kids. Luckily, we had a restroom in our classroom since we were a kindergarten class. After discovering that I have had Asperger's Syndrome and doing some research on it, I now know that all the bathroom training issues were due to the Asperger's itself.

From what I can recall of Kindergarten playing and making "friends" seemed to come easily for me. I put the "friends" in quotations because with a more mature outlook on things now I realize that at that age level making friends isn't really something you have to try to do or work at. It seems like it was staged for us or set up that way by a teacher. I would say that I got kind of close with a couple of kids. Luckily the kid I had mentioned before "Eric" was also in my Kindergarten class. This was back at the time when we had half day Kindergarten, so school didn't become too overwhelming for me or last too long. I can remember the first time I got invited to another kid's birthday party was in the spring or end of the school year in Kindergarten. I was invited to go to Chucky Cheese, which at the time I think may have still been called "Showbiz Pizza." I went up with about three or four other boys and played some of the games and had some pizza. I can't really remember how well the social interaction was for me during that event as it was so early in life, but I do remember just coming home and feeling kind of left out or different. In fact, there were several times during Kindergarten where I started to and did feel different. However, I didn't think anything of it at all.

Now that Kindergarten was officially over with for the year I was ready to move on to the first grade. At least I thought so. I honestly believe that first grade very well could have been where I first really felt different and out of place. Now I had no idea at the time that this was going on or what it was, but I did feel different. In the next chapter you will learn what it was like for me to go through the early elementary years. In chapter two I will discuss grades 1-3 and some of the events that took place within those years. I think these were very crucial years for me. I think this is where most NT's really start to develop the skill set that is necessary to use in the late elementary school and middle school years to develop friendships with other peers.

2 DISTRACTIONS AND DIFFICULTIES

Going from Kindergarten into first grade was quite a significant change for me. Now instead of only being at school for a half day I had to be there for the better of six or seven hours. The entire day! I wasn't sure what to think about this change. I would say that this is where I first noticed that the change of routine thing became difficult for me. During my first-grade year I was somehow able to develop an even better friendship with my friend Eric, in which I had met back in preschool.

Eric and I were always out on the playground together playing game involving running around, hiding, or chasing each other. There were a few other kids that played with us. I can remember that while most of the kids were often running around starting trouble with one another I seemed to be rather quiet and keep to myself as much as I could. Even within the group that I was playing those games with, I often seemed to wonder about by myself and not really fit in with the rest of the group.

Knowing everything that I know now I can look back overall first grade experience and realize that I was spending much of my time alone because I didn't seem to be able to fit in or hangout with the other kids. Even in the classroom I felt like the other kids seemed to know something I didn't about socializing and this really through me for a loop. Of course, I had no idea that there was any meaning behind socializing nor do I think I even knew what the word socializing met, but I know that I could tell that there was just something different about the other kids, or something different about me.

Bullying

First grade was the very first time in my life to where I ever experienced someone being mean to me or teasing me. Now that I'm older I now know that this was something that we often refer to as "bullying." Recently I found a definition in the dictionary about what a bully is. A bully is a blustering, quarrelsome, overbearing person who habitually badgers and intimidates smaller or weaker people. One of the bullies that I most remember is a boy by the name of Stephan. Stephan was kind of a rougher kid who didn't seem to know how to follow the rules set forth in the classroom. No matter what the teacher would ask Stephan to do, he always seemed to end up doing something completely opposite and disrupting the class. There was another bully by the name of Shawn. He was always a big kid who if he wanted to could pretty much scare any kid.

Between these two students I was often made fun of if not a

little bit abused. To this day I'm not sure if it's something that they meant to do or if they were just being themselves and not realizing that they were bothering or hurting someone else. I am someone who likes and needs for things to be quiet. I don't like a lot of loud noises or destructions. Especially when I'm trying to learn. I feel like if there is too much else going on in the room then I'm not able to focus on learning the material that is being presented to me. Of course, after finding out I had Asperger's Syndrome I have now recently begun to understand why this is. We know that people with Asperger's Syndrome will most often struggle with trying to organize things in their brain and focusing in on something when there is more than one thing going on at a time. Let's just say that multitasking is and was never my strong point in life.

So, with a lot of kids not realizing or not understanding the need to be quiet when the teacher or someone else of importance was talking or leading a group discussion I was never able to focus in and learn what was being taught to me. It seemed like a lot of kids just didn't really notice or care that there was a teacher up in front of the classroom trying to do her job and teach the students relevant information that they needed to learn. I was always very puzzled that when the teacher asked us to be quiet that I would always still hear kids whispering to each other if not talking aloud to one another in the classroom. I could never understand this. To me be quiet means exactly that, BE QUIET.

I was very fortunate to have my cousin in the same first

grade class as I was in. I think this was something that really helped me to cope and deal with everything that was going on all at once. My cousin and I had always got along and spent a lot of time together in childhood. We would spend the night at each other's house whenever we could. He would stay at my house more often than I would his due to some circumstances that were beyond our control. We had always got along well with no problems. Unfortunately, there was a day in first grade which was severely tragic to the development of my self-esteem. You see as a kid I had always had trouble with bed wetting and controlling bowel movements. I was actually very surprised but relieved to learn that one of the effects of having Asperger's Syndrome is Bedwetting and bowel movement issues.

Sometimes I would have problems at school. I always hated to ask the teacher if I could get up and leave the classroom as I felt like I was bothering her in some way. To this day I still don't like to interrupt people with a silly question or any question at all. I'm pretty sure that this is due to my having Asperger's Syndrome.

One day in the first grade towards the end of the day I had this horrible experience occur that was again very detrimental in the development of my self-esteem. I remember that we had a substitute that day. I never enjoyed having a substitute teacher as it most likely meant that the flow of my day or routine was going to be interrupted somehow. It's nearly impossible for a substitute to keep a regular teacher's schedule intact exactly down to the moment. Unfortunately, I think we may have missed a

8

restroom break or two during the day and I ended up having an accident or bowel movement in the classroom. I was trying to make it through to the end of the day, but my cousin ended up coming over to me and smelling something. Now my cousin knew I would often have these accidents and he probably suspected that I had an accident. Not only did he just smell it but then he got down on his knees and proceeded to put his nose down near my butt and sniff. Then after doing that he preceded to get the entire class's attention and point out to them that I'd had an accident and then it was all downhill from there. Other kids then got down on the floor and started sniffing and I started crying. Everyone in the class had known that I had an accident and they were really getting a good laugh out of it with each other. Once again, I was singled out and completely embarrassed in front of all my peers. Later that night I went home and felt so low and was completely distressed about the situation. Little did I know how that was just the beginning of a long series of events that would happen to me in my life.

2nd Grade

Somehow, I managed to make it through that horrific accident in first grade and pass. Moving on to second grade. I got a great teacher and to this day she was still one of my favorite teachers. Mrs. Finley was a very great woman. Unfortunately, she had contracted a form of cancer. She was able to make it through the cancer for a couple of years before passing along to be with the Lord in 1998. I learned a lot of things in second grade. We started to learn a little bit more advanced math. I think we might have gotten into some multiplying and dividing towards the end of the year. Math has always been one of my strong points. To this day I am great with numbers. Mental math is something in which I really excel in. For some reason, I'm also able to quickly memorize telephone numbers and birthdays of everyone I know. I now understand that it's a trait of having Asperger's.

Peer relationships in the second grade seemed to be about like they were in the first grade for me. Again, one or two people that I could sort of talk to and hangout with every now and then. Once again Eric was that person that I really grew to like. He was the type of kid who was what I call the "leader of the pack." He seemed to always be the kid that the other students would want to follow around and sort of worship in a way. I often kind of wondered to myself why the other kids liked him more than they did me. Eric always had some creative game to play and often I didn't really understand why we were playing the game we were, but I just knew that I was sort of playing with someone and making it through school.

As far as the bullying goes in the second grade, I think that there were still the same kids that were causing problems in the first grade. Always talking and being a distraction in class and really interfering with me and I'm sure another student's ability to learn. I'm not exactly sure if this is a good thing or not but I seemed to behave more like the girls in the class. For some reason I didn't understand the behavior of my male counterparts. I was more soft and delicate and not wanting to bother anyone or become a distraction. It often seemed to me that boys were just looking to cause trouble or to become the center of attention. I never understood this. (I should note that to this day I still feel like it's easier for me to get close to girls on a friendship level than it is to other guys.) I will explain this in further detail in a later chapter.

Another huge thing that was a problem for me towards the end of second grade involved my sensory motor skills. Towards the very end of second grade I can vaguely remember starting to try and write cursive. Unfortunately for me this was a huge struggle at first. I already knew that I had trouble with penmanship, but I didn't know why at the time. Now I can understand and appreciate that it was due to the late development of my sensory motor skills. I would say that I still have quite a significant amount of trouble with some sensory motor skills. Luckily for me Mrs. Finley was a very patient person and she was always very encouraging. She took the time to practice with me and help me learn how to hold the pencil and write the letters. I can remember tracing letters for hours upon hours. This got a little boring to me and again I really struggled to see the reason or point to us learning how to write letters in a different way. I could not make any sense of it. I think this is another issue that may have caused the other kids to make fun of me.

Third Grade

Third grade was an important year for me. I got lucky and ended up with a great teacher. Mrs. See's was one of my all-time favorite teachers and I was fortunate enough to get lucky to have her twice in Elementary school as she ended up moving up to sixth grade. Schoolwork seemed to come easy to me in that year. That was also the year that things started to heat up at school socially with the peers. This was probably the first time I can recall going to afterschool events with other kids. It was one thing for me to be able to talk to other students during the day, but as I was about to find out it was something totally new and different, something extremely challenging for me, to go to afterschool events and try to socialize with other kids outside of the school day.

Obsessions or Special Interests

I should note that as a kid growing up it was always a goal of mine to become a professional basketball player. (Pretty lofty goal, I know right?) Well in third grade I had a cousin who was in the sixth grade and was playing on the elementary basketball team. I can also remember one of the girls in my class (Sarah Hanson) had an older sister who was on the girls' basketball team. Her name was Kortney, she was the same age as my cousin. So, I started going to all the basketball games as basketball was always my favorite sport. I would often try and sit with Sarah. To this day I don't know if Sarah and I are actually "friends" I mean to me she was always a good friend and extremely nice to me, but we've never really hung out outside of the school day since about fourth grade I think.

As I was watching the basketball games I noticed something very strange about myself. To this day I'm not exactly sure why this was. I was enjoying watching our girls' basketball team a lot more than the boy's team. This could be due to a few reasons, one of which was the girls team could have surely beat our boys team hands down which meant they were winning a lot more games and more fun to watch. I really became interested in the two stars of that team. That would have been the 1994-95 school year. The stars of the team were Kortney, which was Sarah's sister and then a girl by the name of Alexia Shields. Alexia was like Michael Jordan to me. That girl would throw up shots that only MJ would dream of taking and somehow manage to get the roll and have the shot find the bottom of the net. To this day, I can still recall one play and remember exactly what happened. She managed to drive in the lane and draw contact from an opposing player. She got completely turned around and managed to throw up a ridiculous backwards shot while not even looking at the rim and it rolled around up there for a couple seconds but somehow found the bottom of the net. She even got fouled and converted the three-point play.

Now that I've been diagnosed with Asperger's Syndrome I have learned that there are many components that come along with having Asperger's Syndrome. This is a huge reason as to why Asperger's is so easily diagnosed with other disorders. Obsessive Compulsive Disorder or OCD is something that is very common to have when someone has Asperger's Syndrome. Knowing what I know now I can say that Basketball girls' basketball and the individual players in which were talented, and the stars of the team became a fascination to me. I wanted to know everything about them. I wanted to memorize their stats from every game. One of the things in which I've noticed in my life is that I like to talk about things a lot and have often seemed to over talk about things I'm interested in until it gets to the point of driving the other person crazy. I think this happened with Sarah as I would always want to talk to her during the school day about the previous day's basketball game or the upcoming basketball game. I am almost sure she hated me for always bugging her about her sister or the games.

This would also be the year that I started to become very interested in the high school team. The high school (Huntington North) had a very good basketball team was extremely talented that year. Infect that was the year (1994-95) in which they went to state and won their second state title over Lake Central. To this day I'm not sure why I like women's basketball more than men's but it's true that I do enjoy watching a women's game more so than the guys.

As far as the rest of the year in third grade: it seemed to be normal. I really started to notice that groups seemed to be developing. It seemed like people were forming more friendships with other students and congregating in groups more so in the third grade than they seemed to in the previous two or three years of school. I wondered why so and so was hanging out with such and such a group. I was never really included in those groups that would just congregate and stand around chatting about whatever it was they chatted about. I really would have liked to have been but for some reason in which I could not figure out, (and I spent a lot of time just trying to figure out exactly what it was they just didn't really want to include or interact with me. I managed to pass the third grade with flying colors.

Cursive writing was still very much a struggle for me and something that I had to work at extremely hard.

In the next chapters I will discuss in detail my experiences of Fourth-Sixth grade at Andrews Elementary school. It is important to pay attention to and notice how the "game" or concept of socializing among peers seems to change quite a bit within these years as kids are getting older. I would refer to it as just a maturing of the socializing process. As you may know, this is something that people with Asperger's syndrome would struggle with severely. As a side note I would add that if you are a parent of a child in which seems to be having problems coping with school or changes to routines or even behavior that you would have them evaluated as Asperger's and Autism Spectrum disorders are becoming a much more common thing these days. I would say that it's probably due to us having more knowledge and being able to recognize and quickly diagnose those students. I feel that it is crucial for a child to get diagnosed at as early of an age as possible so that they can get the proper help and support that will be needed to succeed not only in social relationships with peers, but as you will soon find out they would also benefit from getting support and help to help them succeed in their academics as well as employment in the future. These concepts will all be discussed in detail in a later chapter.

3 THE LAST KID PICKED

Fourth grade was probably one of my most favorite years in Elementary school. I had the opportunity of having a cool teacher who was fresh out of college. I remember being amazed that this teacher was only 23 years old at the time. I thought wow. He's not that much older than I am. As always it was difficult for me to adjust to the new teacher and the new school year. There would be a lot of new beginnings that year for us fourth graders. Just like in the past, most of these kids were better equipped to handle the challenges of the change.

I remember on the first or second day of school a rather humorous situation. Our teacher, Mr. Graf had taken us outside to read a story and we were gathered around a tree and somehow his pants ripped. The New Year seemed to start off okay and I was just getting back into the flow of things from having the summer off.

Changes in Fourth Grade

I can remember a few changes that seemed to occur in the Fourth Grade. One of the major ones for me was the fact that we were now required to start having gym clothes. So that we could change when we went to gym and then re-change again at the end of gym class. This was a good thing because at about that age I think we all start to sweat and smell after gym. However, it seemed awkward for me. I'm not sure why. Maybe it was because I struggled with tying shoes due to my poor motor skills. Either was I somehow managed to survive changing in the locker rooms.

Another huge change for me was that we were now in the upstairs part of the building. For the first four years of my school career we were downstairs. Three of those years were spent in the new part of the building and we had air conditioning. Now I was upstairs for the remaining three years of Elementary School. For some reason I was never very fond of stairs and this would come back to haunt me within that following year or so. I can recall that I was scared to walk up the stairs due to not knowing if I would be able to stand up or stay on my feet. Then I would see these kids that were taking two steps at a time and everyone thought it was cool. SO, I would think that I needed to take them two at a time, so I could fit in.

The year went well for me as far as school. I generally got all A's during Elementary school. It was an adjustment for me having a male teacher for the first time however. I was worried at first that he would not be able to be as nice or understanding as the female teachers I've had and or not as willing to help. But it turned out that he was very understanding. He would encourage me to do a lot of things and push me to excel.

Organization Skills

I remember that throughout my school career teachers were trying to teach me how to be cleaner and organized as far as school stuff. For example. I often had the habit of just throwing the textbooks and my notebooks back in my desk. I could see the logic in trying to put them in there neatly because I was just going to pull them back out again later. It just didn't make sense to me and I wouldn't have known how to organize them. Now I know that yet again another characteristic of Asperger's is that people with it do not have good organization skills. Now it makes sense to me. So, somehow, I'd always manage to have the messiest desk of any student in the classroom.

One day I was encouraged by Mr. Graf to organize and clean my desk. So, as I tried to clean I was thinking that I would come up with a good system for keeping things neat. I wrote down all my books and where they were going to be at in my desk. I taped this list to my desk. This told me which book was on which side of my desk and what book was on top of what book, so I could just reach in and quickly grab the book I needed without any worries or consuming too much time. I often remember that when the teachers were ready to start a lesson in a new subject I would be searching for my book and they'd end up waiting on me to find my book before they would start the lesson. This was kind of embarrassing to me because this meant that every other student was sitting there staring at me and laughing at me while I was searching for my book.

In my system I did what was logical to me which was probably completely illogical to the other NT's in the room. I abbreviated the first three letters of the subject that the book was about. So, English= ENG. Math=Mat, Science-Sci, and so on. Then a situation I remember occurring is that we had an assignment book in which students are supposed to use to keep them more organized and to make sure they write all their homework down so that they don't miss or forget about an assignment. Well the first three letters of that book were Ass. So, I wrote that down and I didn't think anything of it. Later, another student saw that and pointed it out to the teacher and caused a huge scene. I couldn't figure out why this other student was pointing something out on my desk to a teacher. I hadn't done anything wrong. Well, Mr. Graf had to explain to me why we should change that and make it more appropriate. I would have never even thought of that but maybe it was because I never used foul language. To this day those little things like that still really don't make sense or register in my brain.

Socializing in Fourth Grade

Socializing in Fourth grade was a unique experience to say the least. I noticed that some things were changing about the way in which kids were playing on the playground. No longer were the girls playing babies or something to that nature. No longer were the boys running around chasing each other playing cowboys and Indians. In fact, the boys weren't chasing the boys anymore. They started to chase the girls.

I remember that it seemed like these boys completely did a 180. Throughout my first few years of school it was like the playground was segregated. The boys would do their own thing and then the girls did their own thing. Somewhere along the lines, something happened, and boys and girls became fascinated with each other. Not to an extreme. I believe this was still the point where girls were saying boys had cooties or something. I could never understand that phrase and comment for the life of me. I think I went around asking parents and grandparents what cooties were after hearing that at school the first couple of times.

Eric was still the leader of the pack in my group. It seemed like everywhere he went, we went. Some kids started to play sports at recess. Since I had always loved basketball I would try to play along with the other boys who were playing at recess. I was pretty good but for some reason no one wanted me on their team. Kids do a thing to where they have team captains and the team captains pick the teams. I was always the last kid picked which to me meant I was worthless and only picked by someone because they were forced to pick me. Some kids would swing on the swing set and talk. Talking started to become more of a thing in making friends at this level. It was less play, more talk.

Huntington North Girls Basketball Team

Earlier I had spoken about how in Third grade I an obsession or fascination with girls had that played sports.

Mainly girls that played basketball. The Huntington North Lady Vikes won that Indiana state basketball championship in 1995. I watched those state finals games on television. The 1995-96 season promised to be a great season with the possibility of repeating. The girls were remarkable this year. I remember my parents taking me to almost every game. They quickly became nationally ranked as they were already the number one team in Indiana. I can't remember what they were for sure, but I think they may have been as high as the number two team in the nation.

There were several good players on that basketball team; however, my favorite was a girl by the name of Lisa Winter. Lisa was a very beautiful girl and she was extremely talented with a basketball. I became fascinated by Lisa and I remember trying to sit as close to the team bench in every game just hoping that she'd say hi to me. Lisa would later go on to be named Miss Basketball for the state of Indiana in 1996.

The team cruised to an undefeated regular season and I was super excited about the tournament. Back then when it was still "Hoosier Hysteria" the tournament was a breeze for us at Huntington North. We would play small schools in the sectional and blow them out. We would rarely see a worthy opponent until the championship game of the Regional or Semi-State. We ended up running into a very worthy and determined opponent in the semi-state championship game that year. Kokamo High school would upset the Lady Vikes. I remember being so sad because we had tickets to the state finals the Saturday after at Market Square Arena in Indianapolis. Nevertheless, I was totally into Lisa and just wanted to meet her. I have no idea what she's doing now but to this day I would still really enjoy meeting her and I would love to shoot hoops with her or play her one on one.

At that time, it wasn't really an "oh my gosh" she's hot thing for me. It was just like she was more of a role model. I'm not sure why this was. Again, I attribute it to the fact that I've always thought girls were nicer than boys and I would tend to get along with them better because they were more understanding. Looking back on it now I guess you could say that she was something that brightened my day and gave me something to look forward to whenever I could go see a basketball game at the high school. Thanks Lisa!

5th Grade "The big and tragic change #1

5th grade would prove to be a significant year for me. I had a great teacher and still excelled academically but something happened in October. I remember exactly how it went down. Eric Miller, the only kid that I was kind of friends with told us while sitting on a swing set that his dad had got a job in Cedar Rapids, Iowa and the family was moving away. I was stunned. I couldn't believe this was happening. I think this kind of set me back in some ways. We spent the next month enjoying all the time we had left together and then we had to say our goodbyes and part ways. I really struggled with this. Luckily my teacher was aware of the situation and quickly acted to ensure that I made another friend I could count on. Mrs. Ross was understanding and a good teacher. For some reason I remember that her teaching style was easiest for me to handle.

Somehow, I ended up being friends with Austin Davenport. Austin was completely different than Eric. More adventurous. We did different types of things like play basketball and I guess you could say more athletic stuff. We seemed to get along well and would start to do some things outside of school. We would attend high school basketball games and hangout at each other's houses.

5th grade was very exciting to me as we had a new basketball coach, and this was the first year that I could play elementary basketball. I didn't start that year, but I played in quite a few games and took a few shots. The sixth graders were decent that year and we had a good time. I remember us playing and going all the way to the Semifinals of the county tournament in which Central Elementary beat us by a final score of 34-31. I really enjoyed the year of basketball and was looking forward to the next year with Mr. Ginder as a coach. He seemed to have a good understanding of basketball and how to teach it.

The survived the rest of fifth grade managing to get good grades and get by socially. 5th grade would also be the year that a major change at home was about to take place. I grew up as an only child, but I had always wanted a brother or sister. Someone to play with more often. Well one day when I was in fifth grade my mom tells me she's pregnant. Quite a shock to me. I was going to finally have a sibling. I was very excited. I wasn't sure how to handle the change though.

Boys Interest in Girls.

As I touched on earlier it was about this time that something strange was happening in social relationships. Boys were starting to become fond of girls. I remember now watching them interact with each other with little or no interest of girls at the time. Meaning I didn't think about it or wonder about it as much as the other boys did. Now as I look back on this often I wonder if maybe that isn't the reason in which I struggle with dating so much now. I think maybe I should have been more interested at the time. I can recall my cousin Dusty, whom I mentioned earlier in this book was one of these boys that was crazy about girls. There was one girl he seemed to for a liking to. Her name was Shellie Vigored. Shellie was and still is a very attractive girl. But even thinking back now, I can recall going back to third grade how Dusty would talk and talk and talk to these girls for a long time. Especially Shellie. I would always wonder up to his house at night after school and he'd be talking on the phone forever before he would come out. At that point in time I had no interest in girls nor did I have an interest in chatting it up with a girl or anyone for that matter on the phone. Talking wasn't my forte. I just never knew what to say. Now if only my lack of interest in girls would have stayed that way. Boy it sure didn't. More about this later.

4 JUST PASSING THROUGH

Getting into the beginning of the sixth-grade year was an exciting opportunity for me. I was glad to be excelling through school and was glad to have the friendship with Austen to replace that of what was lost when Eric and his family moved away. No friendship can be replaced but I think that have another friend or someone to talk to can help lessen the pain of losing a friend to a move.

I had Mrs. See's again for my sixth-grade year. There was also something a little different about sixth grade. In sixth grade we had two teachers. We had a teacher who would teach us for one period of the day that was not our regular classroom teacher. I couldn't understand this change for the life of me. Why would I need two teachers to teach me school stuff? None the less that's how it happened. For me this was very difficult. I had trouble adapting to the fact that each of these teachers seemed to have a completely different teaching style that stumped me. I mean I was used to Mrs. See's teaching style but when I went over to learn about Science I was not equipped to handle the style of Mr. Winter. Also, I think again having the contrast of having a female and a male teacher at the sometime was a difficult concept for me. Teaching styles are just so much different and their ability to be understanding and caring sometimes isn't quite the same. Some male teacher's I've had have been wonderful in explaining things. However, a lot of them would just give an assignment and then expect you to be able to start and complete it without needing any help. I did survive the year academically however I think I managed to receive my first C. This was the first time that school was a little bit of a challenge to me. My handwriting was improving a little. (It was still nowhere close to being neat.) I was learning and grasping the concept of writing in cursive finally.

Cross Country Experience

In fifth and sixth grade I had the opportunity to participate on our cross-country teams. To this day I'm not sure exactly why I decided to join that team, but I think I somehow managed to take something away from it. I was a terribly slow runner and completely uncoordinated. (I now run three miles per day with ease.) Every race in which we had I would finish near the back of the pack. I was always the last runner from our school to finish any race. After being last repeatedly, it kind of put me down and I just didn't think I was any good. I mean yeah, I finished the race, but the other kids were already off celebrating finishing and running off without me. Now that I look back on it I feel great about just finishing every race because running was very hard for me. I think I joined because I thought it would be a great opportunity for me to meet people and try and make friends.

Basketball Season

Basketball was and has always been my favorite sport. I played a little in fifth grade but didn't see a whole lot of game action. 6th grade promised to be an exciting year for me as I was one of the tallest and biggest kids to be on the team. We had a new coach take over as Mr. Ginder would depart after teaching just one year at Andrews Elementary. Mr. Winter would be the new coach and he definitely had a unique coaching style. His style was totally different than that of Mr. Ginder.

I remember being so excited about basketball. The only thing I hated about basketball was that we had to do a lot of running that didn't even have anything to do with basketball. I could never understand why it was necessary to run up and down the stairs so many times and waste about an hour of practice just running. Our team only won one game that year as we struggled to understand our roles on the team.

Somehow during the year, the other boys on the team gave me an "unwanted" nickname. They came up with the idea for calling me the "Beef." I guess this was because I was bigger than the rest of the team and now I'm sure they meant no harm with their statements. Saying something like that to a kid whom already has a low self-esteem can be detrimental.

I made it through basketball season that year, but it was very frustrating. I had originally won the starting center position. After two games the coach pulled me aside to let me know that I wouldn't be starting anymore because I wasn't fast enough. I was really discouraged, and I remember I wanted to quit. Everyone would always make fun of me when we ran because I ran weird and extremely slow. I managed to gut it out and finish out the year.

Memorable play and experience

I will always remember a play that happened during our first basketball game of the year in sixth grade. We were playing a much more athletically talented team than we were, and we had fallen behind 8-0. After falling behind, we tried to run a play and it got broken up. The point guard who was my cousin Dusty ended up driving into the lane and drawling my man off me. I was wide open and somehow Dusty was able to get the ball to me. I shot it and swooshed it nothing but net. I was kind of amazed but nevertheless we were on the scoreboard. I will always remember that play for as long as I live as it is something that I can feel good about.

Discovering a Passion which would later turn into the "Special Interest"

In sixth grade we would be offered a chance to join the band. I was always more interested in athletics than anything else in the world and had never been interested in joining the band. However, my cousin Dusty was pumped to join the band and play the drums. He talked me into joining as well. Little did I know at the time just how important this decision would be for me as it would later turn into a unique opportunity for a career.

So here we were. Instrument fitting night. I didn't really have any interest in playing percussion, so I was looking at other sections in the band to try out. I was fond of the trumpet, so I tried to play the trumpet, but it was extremely difficult. It turns out that my mouth was just too big for the trumpet. So, the next instrument that was handed to me was a trombone. Well this was an interesting instrument to me because unlike any other instrument the notes could be played by moving a slide. I thought "Wow, this is something unique and I can handle this." I played it and quickly fell in love with it.

We would have many opportunities to present concerts that first year. Mr. Campbell was the band teacher. We learned how to play together and make music. I would quickly become fascinated in the trombone and the noises that you could make with it. I started taking it home and practicing literally every day. I decided that I wanted to become a master at the instrument.

Carrying on about the "Special Interest" for too long.

Often people with Asperger's Syndrome will become obsessed with their special interest. Sometimes we tend to carry on and on about it for too long. I remember that in sixth grade there was a time when our girls' team got beat. Our girl's teams were good, so this didn't happen very often. But one of the girls on the team, Sarah Hanson, whom I mentioned before got injured in one of those games.

The next day following the game in school somehow, I ended up talking about the game that took place the night before with Sarah. I remember her getting upset and saying that she didn't want to talk about it anymore. She then proceeded to tell several other kids that I was bugging her by going on and on about the game. I felt bad that I had hurt her in some way, but I didn't understand what I was doing wrong or what could be so hurtful about talking about a game from the night before.

Of course, I now know that us Aspie's can carry on and on about our special interest. Special interests are things that people whom have an autistic diagnosis become obsessed with. This is something that we become obsessed with more so than a normal interest. The intensity level of the interest is much greater than that of a "normal" interest if indeed there really is such a thing as normal.

With not being able to understand social communication and context of the social situations we are in its extremely easy for us to get talking about our special interest and then not be able to get off the topic. This is problematic as people tend to see us as being rude or overbearing. This is completely unintentional by the person with Asperger's.

There are many reasons for why this happens. For me one of the reasons is because I don't understand social communication at all. To me when I am socializing in someone I feel like I am dumb and from a different world. You feel all alone, and you don't know how to initiate a conversation with anyone. Because of not knowing how to initiate a conversation and not knowing what to talk about with others, I get nervous and anxious. It is simple to talk about something I am interested in and know practically everything about. Because I don't know what else to say I tend to talk about my special interests. I am not trying to be rude by doing this, but I don't know what else to say. Or more appropriately, I don't know how to say what I want to say.

Sixth Grade Graduation

Well, it was June of 1998 and I was done with elementary school. I was ready to move onto the next chapter of my life. This next area of life would be one that was challenging for me. It was full of many changes. Changes that I had a difficult time adapting to. I was ready for Jr. High or middle school.

Jr. High is a crucial time for everyone. NT's and Aspie's alike having to go through so many changes and adapt to so many different things. Puberty kicks in and changes start happening to our bodies and without proper knowledge and understanding this can be really depressing for individuals. People on the Autism spectrum tend to have a much more difficult time in handling puberty.

Changes in how friendships work

To me, this is the area that was of significance. In middle school the way kids socialize with each other changes. Throughout elementary school kids would socialize by running around on the playground chasing each other. Or playing silly games. As we get older we start to base our friendships more on conversations. If you have any understanding of autism at all you know how difficult that conversation is and can quickly see why this would be such a challenging time.

Also, middle school is a crucial time when the self-esteem really blossoms and develops. Without proper friendships and support someone on the spectrum will not be able to develop a good self-esteem. As I have stated before, I think it's extremely important that if you notice anything thing about your child that makes you think or throws you for a loop that you should take him or her to see someone. The quicker you get a diagnosis, the better off you will be. I cannot stress that point enough. I know myself that I would have benefited greatly by being diagnosed at an elementary age as opposed to not finding out until I was 22. I will be talking about a good "indicator" that someone could have an Autistic disorder in the next chapter. This is extremely important. However, like any diagnosis, it's hard to determine if this is just a NT going through a rough transition or if it's a child struggling because he or she is autistic.

5 FAILING SOCIALIZING

Seventh grade was a learning experience for me. It was like nothing I had ever experienced before. I was going to a new school which was a lot bigger than my elementary school. I would have to meet new teachers. I would also have to meet new students as kids from other elementary schools would be going to the same middle school as I did.

All of this was a lot to handle. I remember the first day of school I was terrified. Seventh grade presented many challenges for me and it was also the first year that I can remember having some difficulty with academics. I had done poorly in penmanship before, but I'd never struggled in any other subject.

At Riverview Middle School each grade was split up into two teams. I think they called them the Red and Gold teams. I believe I was on the gold team in Seventh Grade. Each team had four teachers that would teach the main academic subjects of Math, Science, Social Studies, and English. Then we would have about two to three other teachers who taught either band/choir, Physical Education, or Keyboarding. There was also a teacher to teach a subject called Industrial Technology or something to that affect.

I could never ever see the point in us having to take Industrial technology and in fact, I hated it. I think it was because I was not very skilled at building or making things. With the sensory problems I have always found it difficult to build things with my hands. Other people seem to be able to put things together with no problem, but for me it's a real struggle and it often gets frustrating.

I remember how the other kids would just sit and point while laughing at me. Then often whoever was teaching the class would get frustrated and to me it seemed like they thought that I wasn't trying. However, I was trying hard. Often, I felt like people just hated me. I couldn't see why they couldn't understand me.

The Core Subjects in teams

Each team would have four academic subjects each day. We would be on a rotation with the same people. So at least the students in the class were always the same and new each other. Now that I can look back on this from an educated prospective I would say that Seventh grade was the year to where I really felt out of place and like something was wrong with me. However, I didn't speak to anyone about feeling this way until years later. I would have benefited if I would have talked to someone about the way I felt years before I did.

Therefore, I would suggest to parents of all students. That you actively engage in your child's education. Not just helping them with the academics but asking them to make sure everything is going okay for them and making sure they are adjusting to changes properly. Change is something that can be extremely challenging to deal with for anyone. Even some adults have some difficulty accepting change. People who are on the spectrum live by a routine. Anything that interrupts that routine can cause severe discomfort.

It was during each of these core subjects that I would try so hard to make friends and get to know people. For some reason other kids would generally always be talking with each other in our free time. A lot of students would be laughing and enjoying each other's company. Rather it be socializing or gossiping they all seemed to be engaged in conversation. I wanted to be involved in their conversations so badly, but I was scared to try. When I did muster up the courage to attempt to join in a conversation with a classmate or a group of classmates it went terrible. It was always a horrifying experience to me and very damaging to my self-esteem.

The middle school years are also very crucial in the development of the self-esteem. These middle school years are often the years that kids become friends in groups. Clicks tend to form and if you're not in the "in crowd" you really know about it.

My First Locker

I remember getting my first locker in Seventh Grade. I was such a mess because I was afraid I wasn't going to be able to remember the combination or get it opened. However, that was not the case at all as I can still remember the combination to this day. 19-25-21. however, I would end up not enjoying the locker scene so much due to some other circumstances.

I probably don't have to tell you that my locker ended up becoming a very unorganized filing cabinet. Organization of supplies is something I still struggle with to this day. Now if it's keeping dates organized I'm your man as I remember nearly everything. But I would have papers everywhere as well as books. I am surprised that I was able to find the correct book at the time when I needed it.

Another problem that I had with the lockers is that other kids would want to socialize near them before school, in between passing periods and then again after school. It seems like these kids were doing nothing but talking to one another all day long. To this day I can't understand how they did it. How did they know what to say to each other? I would often think (and to this day) still think that someone has handed this kids and adults even a book that tells them what to talk about. I believe that I am missing that book and that it is the key to developing successful social relationships with people.

The problem in this was not only the fact that I quickly became frustrated when I saw what was going on. I could see them there socializing with each other and talking about stuff. The stuff I am referring to is what NT's would refer to as "Small Talk." This seemed to be something that other kids did with little or no effort at all. On top of this, several people would congregate around my locker to socialize with other students who had lockers near me but were so much more popular than I was and ever would become. So, with everyone often crowding around my locker I couldn't get to it when I needed to sometimes. I can recall several occasions in which I went to go get something from my locker or return something to my locker in which there would be anywhere from five to ten people standing in front of my locker just chit chatting. There were often when I would need to get a book out of the locker to take to a class. Well I would stand around waiting for the students to go away but it seemed like they never did. Eventually I would give up and just go on to class without the materials that I needed because I didn't want to bother them by trying to get something from my locker. Honestly, I don't think I knew how to interrupt them so that I could say what I needed to say. There were also plenty of nights in which I wouldn't want to go to my locker after school. Not because I didn't want to in fact I needed to but because there were once again people standing around my locker and blocking it from me. I felt as if my own locker was off limits to me and that other kids were using it. Often, I would go home without a jacket or coat because of this.

I remember constantly wanting to be the first student to arrive at school in the morning. I panicked if the bus was running late or didn't get us to school on time. I wanted to be the first student in the building so that I could just go to my locker and get what I needed. Sometimes I would try to carry around extra stuff for two or three class periods because I knew that I would have no chance of getting to my locker during the day. I didn't do this because I wanted to but because I felt like I had to. Even if on a rare occasion I did get to my locker I didn't want to take the time because I wanted to be the first person in the classroom to pick a seat. If I picked my seat, then if another student had to sit beside me it was because they chose to or were the last one in the room. I always would feel bad if I would be late and try to sit next to someone. I would feel like I was hurting them because they didn't like me and that I didn't belong in the class with the other students.

Socializing and the Movies

I recall that I noticed in Seventh grade how other kids would not only socialize with more success than I did at school, but their friendships started to go outside of school as well. Huntington was just opening a new movie theatre called the Huntington Seven. Now this was unique to Huntington because before this the theatre was downtown and only one screen.

Well what ended up happening is that kids now had somewhere to hangout and socialize outside of school. Kids would be at the movies every Friday night with their friends. These friendships seemed to come in numbers now like I'd never seen before. Meaning it seemed to me as if there were certain kinds of kids hanging out with each other in groups. During the school day and then again outside of school people would congregate in groups of people. This was extremely uncomfortable for me as I was never a part of a group and left to wonder around by myself. These groups of kids would be at the movies on a Friday night with their friends not their parents. I know this because when I was at the movies with my parents I would see them all there congregating outside of the theatre with each other and having amazing social interactions. I became frustrated and tried to avoid going to the movies as much as possible.

Feelings and emotions

I can tell you that this was the year in which I really started to become bothered by the fact that I felt different and that other kids seemed "cooler" and more popular to me at that time. Unfortunately for me I didn't think too much of it at the time other than to myself. I became down on myself at times and thought I was stupid. I didn't understand why I had such a hard time. Now luckily for me I would end up having what I now refer to as a "coping" mechanism.

Coping Mechanism and 7th Grade Band

Along with the transition to a new school came a new band director or teacher. Mr. Michael Flanagan was the band instructor at Riverview Middle School. The middle schools in Huntington had a summer band program so my summer between the sixth and seventh grade came to an end a couple of weeks early. I remember the seventh-grade year that both middle schools had the summer band program at Riverview because Crestview middle school was transitioning into their new building and it was not quite ready for them.

This was a unique experience for me. In sixth grade we only had around ten to thirteen people in the band. Well now, with all the elementary schools going to the middle school we would have a band of around fifty instrumentalists. I ended up really enjoying the summer band program that year. I had such a great time and the best part was that I had fun without having to socialize with anyone or trying to make friends. Trying to make friends is extremely painful for me. So, I guess you could say this experience was kind of a relief for me at the time. I remember that since Crestview was at our school that year we did a combined song called "La Bamba" at the end of the summer program. When the school year started we had to play for Mr. Flanagin as an audition process. Unlike sixth grade this time around we were placed in our sections by talent level.

I would win the position of section leader for the trombones. I was thrilled with this and this gave me something to feel good about as things that made me feel good came far and few between. Being a part of the band at Riverview was a really great experience for me. Without it I think I would have become more depressed and secluded. We quickly prepared for concerts.

As I mentioned before one of my special interests is music. Even at that time I can say that it was a special interest of mine. I loved to play the trombone and was very passionate about it. I can recall several songs that we did. One of them is one of my favorite songs to this day. It is done by the "Canadian Brass" but even as a Seventh-Grade band we were able to perform Pachabell's Cannon. I fell in love with the tune even though it wasn't difficult at all. If you know anything about the song you know that the low brass does not have a very exciting nor challenging part.

We would do other songs like "Castlewood Fantasy." We did a piece for contest named "Pueblo." I can recall several more songs from the 8th grade year that we performed. In 8th grade we were starting to get good. Again, I would be the trombone section leader. We did a lot of songs that year. One was called "Castlerock." We did a piece called "Cumberland Cross" that was a new piece out for band. A lot of the pieces were performing were high school level pieces. I was completely fascinated with music and band. We also performed "The Nutcracker" our Christmas concert.

It was during band that I found an attraction to girls who were good musicians and near the front of their section in rank. I'm not sure what my fascination was but it had to do with a beautiful girl being good at something I was also good at. Maybe a common interest.

Jazz Band

Middle school is a time when students are presented with interesting opportunities. There are clubs and other afterschool programs. Even in the music department there are extracurricular activities for students to get involved in. The opportunities are provided to give students a taste of what it's like at the next level. So, the opportunity came around for me to join the Riverview Jazz Ensemble which was open to both seventh and eighth graders. I debated if I should audition or not. At the time I was still very incompetent in myself socially and musically. I knew that I enjoyed playing trombone though. It was like a way to escape all the horrible things that were happening at school and have some good feelings for a change. So, I took the chance and auditioned and I'm glad I did.

We played a lot of cool stuff in jazz band. I also enjoyed it because this was a completely different type of music. More upbeat. At that point in time in my life being so young I wasn't too thrilled by the classical music we played in concert band, but I loved what we were playing in Jazz Band. We performed pieces called "Louie, Louie" "Rock This Town" "Leader of the Pack" The James Bond Theme Song" "Crazy Little Thing Called Love" "Satin Doll" "Make Me Smile" and 25 or 6 to 4 along with many other great tunes.

Now you're probably wondering why I'm telling you every single song that I've performed in band. Well you're lucky, I haven't even begun to tell you every song in which I've performed, and I'll try not to. But I listed these songs out for you to prove a very valid point. As I've mentioned before people on the spectrum tend to have special interests. These interests can often be more intense than a normal interest. For example, an NT would develop an interest to nearly the same level as an individual on the spectrum. There are other people who have played in these instrumental ensembles with me in the past who I would guess couldn't tell you a single song that we performed way back in the seventh and eighth grade. I can pretty much tell you every single song I've ever played as a musician and who wrote it, when it was written, and who arranged it. As you can see it's easy for someone on the spectrum to go on and on about their interests.

Using the Trombone or Special Interest as a Coping Mechanism

Being as into music as I was and having little or no friends at all I quickly became fascinated by the trombone. I had a good role model as a teacher as Mr. Flanagin was a cool teacher who cared a lot about his students and was very passionate about music. Without the skills to socialize with others I quickly became fascinated with the trombone and would bring it home every night. My parents seemed to enjoy the music, but I don't think they enjoyed me practicing quite so much at home. We live in a small house and it could get loud in there. I would practice about 2-4 hours a night which for a seventh grader is a long time.

In middle school we had practice logs in which we had to fill out on a weekly basis and then return to school for Mr. Flanagin to check. I remember being the student who practiced the most hours of any several times. As much as I really wanted to be like the other kids for some reason I knew I was not. This was really depressing but for someone reason the trombone made it a little easier. Communicating through the trombone and through music was much easier and much more fulfilling for me than trying to socialize with my peers and build friendships and it was a lot less painful.

I would eventually use trombone and music as an even bigger coping mechanism in the years to come. Then a sequence of tragic events pretty much changed my life forever. I will cover this in greater detail in the coming chapters.

Riding the Bus, What a drag!

For me, one of the most horrifying experiences of middle school was riding the bus to and from school. I can't believe how rude kids can be and just how much trouble they can cause. I would get picked up early in the morning by my bus driver and then must change buses at the elementary school in Andrews to get on another bus that was going to Riverview Middle School. The first bus was okay in the morning as there weren't too many kids on it. I wish that bus would have taken us to Riverview instead of having to go through the hassle of switching buses. My bus to Riverview was like a horror film. People would wod up spitballs and throw them all over the place. It was such a disaster. The bus driver couldn't even really focus on driving. It was so loud on there that it was overwhelming for me. I just wanted a calm and peaceful ride to and from school but wow, was that ever hard to get. I think overall, I would say that the bus rides were very dangerous to me because the bus driver had absolutely no control at all. People would throw stuff and hit me. Sometimes people would be verbally abusive or mean to me. They would tease or bully me. Tell me where I could or couldn't sit. It was like a nightmare for me. I was scared. But again, I didn't say anything to anyone not even my parents as I was starting to suspect that the way I was getting treated was the way I was supposed to be treated.

Seventh Grade Basketball Tryouts

Like always I was very into basketball and I decided to try out for the seventh-grade team. I attended the first night of tryouts and completely felt unwelcome and out of place. The other kids wouldn't even acknowledge that I was there. I felt so lonely and lost. This was also about the same time that the jazz band tryouts were taking place and I knew I'd have to decide between doing one or the other anyways. I felt more comfortable in the band room then I did on the basketball court. That first night of basketball tryouts was miserable. Not only did I not fit in socially I just realized that I wasn't nearly as good as these other guys as I was just too slow. I was kind of frustrated about this at the time as I didn't yet know just how good of an experience jazz band would be for me.

Losing the Dream, the first time.

As I have discussed earlier in the book. My dream as a very little kid was to become a professional basketball player in the NBA. It was during my seventh-grade year when I attended basketball tryouts for the very first time that I began to realize that my dream was going to be just that. I didn't have the motor skills or the speed to keep up with the other kids and I wasn't going to cut it at basketball. I was really discouraged for a few weeks. Luckily jazz band would soon get started up and once again, music was a coping mechanism for me. It was at that point in time when the dream switched for me. I gave up on becoming a professional basketball player and decided I'd like to be a professional musician or music teacher. To this day I think that was the best decision I've ever made. Music is so rewarding in so many ways and it comes naturally for me. While I was depressed about losing the dream of becoming a basketball player I am glad that another opportunity was opened for me. In the next chapter we will cover the summer in between my seventh and eighth grade year. We'll then proceed to cover my eight-grade year at Riverview middle school.

6 ESCAPE INTO FANTASYLAND

In between my seventh and eighth grade year I found out something that would be of importance to me. This is something that often happens to an individual who has Asperger's syndrome or autism. I would use this as a coping mechanism for years to come as well.

What I am going to talk about is something that Tony Attwood refers to as "Escape into Imagination" in his book "The Complete Guide to Asperger's Syndrome." Escape into imagination is not just your typical child or adult imagining something. This is much more intense for someone who's on the spectrum. Not only is it more intense but it can also become meaningful to the person.

Just like the special interest having the capability of becoming the individual's best friend, escaping into imagination or a "make believe world" as I like to call it can also become the individual's best friend. Now this is something that is alright in my opinion until it becomes the only means of survival for the individual. If this becomes their life, then we've got a problem.

For me this has been an issue for many times in my life. But at this time, I would escape into the imagination of movies and television shows. During that summer my family had prescribed to receive HBO from Dish Network. While having HBO, I started watching more and more television. I would start watching the movies they'd have on there. I started to become interested in television more and more daily. While I was still playing my trombone quite a bit I was spending the rest of my day watching movies on HBO.

I remember that I would search through the guide to try and find a movie. For some reason, what I was looking for was a movie to where a beautiful woman would be kidnapped. For some reason I was drawn to these movies at the time. I loved the idea of being the "super hero" who comes in and saves the beautiful princess. I came across a wonderful movie that was on HBO one day. This movie would end up airing many times on HBO that summer and I watched it repeatedly. The movie description looked very interesting to me when I read it, so I decided to tape the movie as well. Soon after, I started taping every movie so that I could have a library of movies. (This was something that I did because I wanted to have someone to connect with whenever I wanted.) Again, I think like with everything else I've mentioned, this would be a way of making friends for me. I was unable to make friends in the real world so now I was off to a make-believe world to try and make these friends.

The movie was "Head Above Water." Cameron Diaz is the

main star of this movie and her character is Natalie. Below is a description of the movie. Cameron was great in this movie and I quickly fell in love and became obsessed with her. She's beautiful.

I loved Cameron because she was so funny and attractive. She also had a nice tan and to this day I love women with tans. I was really drawn to Natalie's arms in the movie. I don't know why. This is probably one of the strange special interest I had, but to this day I'm still really drawn to how beautiful a girl's arms are. Anyway, I remember it didn't take long until Natalie would become my best friend. This is probably hard for NT's to understand but when you don't have friends in real life, I think it becomes easy to become creative. This was great for me because this was something that provided meaning for me at that time in my life. Natalie was my best friend and I would imagine every time I watched the movie that I was her hero and saving her.

There is a great scene in the movie where the guy puts Natalie in a bucket of cement or something and then proceeds to dump her into the ocean or a big lake. I remember wishing that I was there to save the day. I would have dived into the water and pulled her to safety. Natalie was amazing to me and I was extremely fascinated by her. I remember wishing that I could meet her in real life.

After that I would watch any Cameron Diaz movie that came out. I have most of them on video. So, you can probably imagine that I was and am also obsessed with the two Charlie's Angels movies. Something about her just makes me happy. She would talk, I could talk to her sort of. But I didn't have to worry at all what she thought about me. To this day she's one of my favorite actresses, I know have a few others, but I still want to meet her someday. It would be like meeting my best friend in the entire world.

I also became more fascinated with television shows such as Saved by the Bell and Full House. For some reason these shows were very appealing to me. Again, I formed a special relationship with the characters with Zack Morris becoming the only guy that I ever became friends with on television. As I've mentioned earlier in the book, I don't even try to make friends with guys anymore as I know that I will just get made fun of, laughed at, beat around, tossed around like a yo yo, or taken advantage of. I will talk more about Zack and Slater from Saved by the Bell in a later chapter when I get into more detail about imitation and escape into imagination. I would later try and imitate how Zack and Slater acted around Kelly and Jessie to try and get girls to like me in real life.

The Beginning of Eighth Grade

The summer of 1999 was pretty laid back for me as I didn't do much of anything at all outside of my fake world. I went swimming on a couple occasions but mostly the only people I saw were my parents and sister and some extended family. After finding a new best friend and having a best friend for the first time in about a year and a half, I'd be excited to start school as I thought maybe it would be easier for me now that I had "Natalie" as the new best friend. If I was going to have a bad day I'd be able to go home and have Natalie get me through it. There were two things which got me through eighth grade. Natalie and band. Once again, I was excited for the summer band program. The seventh-grade band I was in was talented and it promised to be a talented eighth grade band as well. Once again, I would be named section leader of the trombone section. I was extremely excited again and practiced every day. There would be a time in 8th grade where a student by the name of Jeremy would challenge me for my position. I had been challenged before but had always won with ease. This time though Jeremy had won the challenge and played a little better than I had. That was a huge wake up call to me. Now that I look back on it that would have been one of those signs that I was getting to involved with my make-believe world at home. My grades would also start to drop, and school became more challenging for me.

Knowing what I know now, I was escaping into imagination a little too much at home that summer and even during most of my eighth-grade year. I had eased up on the practicing and focused more upon the make-believe world that I had created. I was devastated after losing the challenge because being first chair and section leader was something that I was very proud of and extremely excited about. I moped around for a few days after that, but I immediately started taking my trombone home again and practicing as much as four to five hours a night. I was determined to get my position back and as soon as I was presented the opportunity to do so I would jump on it. I ended up winning my position back and never lost it again after that.

Something else that I'd like to mention is the transition

process from Elementary school to middle school. This can be a complicated transition for anyone but especially for an autistic individual. People on the spectrum become very accustomed to their routines. Disturbing their routines can cause a significant amount of stress.

Going from Elementary school to middle school provides a few things that would change up the routine of the individual and create that stress. One of the biggest and most crucial things is going from having one teacher for your academic subjects all day long to having as many as four to seven teachers throughout each day. This was confusing for me and could be confusing for any individual on the spectrum as well. I would say that the level in which the individual on the spectrum is impacted by these changes depends on the individual themselves. I know that a lot of people have what seems like a stereotype of what Autism is and as soon as they hear that someone they know has autism they immediately start stereotyping and judging the person in what seems like negative and un fair ways. For some reasons our society is one that is quick to stereotype and judge about everything, not just in the field of autism.

It is extremely valuable and important that we keep in mind that just because an individual is autistic it doesn't mean that they aren't a person. There is still a person with feelings and emotions on the inside. A lot of times the individual just doesn't understand or know how to express those feelings and emotions in appropriate ways like NT's do. Basically, it's impossible to say that all people who are autistic have the same characteristics. Rather I would argue that they may share a lot of similar traits, but they also have some things that are unique to themselves such as their special interests.

Most individuals I've met or known on the spectrum do not all have the same special interest. I would bet that if you were standing in a room full of 100 autistic individuals that you wouldn't find two people who had the same special interests. I guess this is my plea to society. Please don't judge people of any type or any illness. Try and understand the person before you make a judgment about them.

Mr. Richison's 8th grade history class.

Mr. Richison was our 8th grade history teacher and he was a very stern man. I ended up really liking him, but I remember for those first few days I was just a little scared of him. I would be put into a cluster with a group of students that included my cousin and a girl by the name of Amy Best. Amy was by far the hottest girl in the eighth grade and I wanted to talk to her so badly. However, I could never ever really develop a great conversation with her and to this day I still haven't been able to develop one.

This class in eighth grade is where I noticed that there was something severely wrong with me. As we sat in the cluster of four people, the other three always had a big social interaction and were connecting with each other sharing laughs and enjoying each other's company. For some reason which was still unknown to me at the time, I could never get myself included in the conversation. I did try on a few occasions and when I would jump in the conversation I remember sometimes getting a strange look and sometimes being ignored like I wasn't even there. This was frustrating for me. Luckily, I had the make-believe world I had created and would often escape into imagination in class while they were having an amazing social conversation.

It was at this time that I really started to feel like there was something wrong with me. Something didn't make sense. I hadn't figured it out yet, nor did I tell anyone I felt this way. It would be many years before I would even talk to anyone about this and then a year or so later before I would be diagnosed.

Eighth Grade Band

Eighth grade band was another exciting year as we would perform many outstanding pieces. Yes, I can tell you just about every piece that we performed that year, but I will spare you and only tell you about one. Because we had such a great trombone section we were able to perform a piece called "Lassus Trombones." This was the most amazing thing to me as it involved playing extremely loud and fast which is something I was very good at. We took the piece to contest and did well as I recall. The thing is I can tell you the notes and rhythms to the song. In fact, it's like I have a library in my head of each song I've ever performed. It's wonderful as I don't even have to have the piece of music in front of me sometimes to perform. I'm not sure if this was due to me having Asperger's syndrome and the fact that music and trombone were special interests of mine or not. I do know that I really enjoy the gift of music that God's given me and intend on using it again sometime here soon.

Band was kind of a fantasy land for me in a way to. I mean it was real. We were playing real notes and making music, but it was done through pushing air through instruments and banging drum heads. The only way anyone could talk was if they were a percussionist and they often did. That is why it was kind of a make-believe world for me because I was communicating through music and not by trying to withhold a conversation with someone. It was relaxing, and I was free. Because I often had the music memorized that we were playing and performing came easily to me I was able to play my part and still be in a dream in my head. I would dream often of being a conductor of an orchestra or performing for a professional orchestra. I am still pursuing these dreams to this day. They were put on hold for a while due to unfortunate circumstances in which I will discuss in a later chapter.

Jazz Ensemble

Jazz band would once again prove to be a positive experience in the eighth grade. We would play many interesting pieces and for the first time in my life we would do a song that had a trombone solo in it. I remember the piece "Over the Rainbow" Everyone's familiar with it. I played the solo enjoyed it. I practiced that solo repeatedly for a few weeks. I wanted it to be perfect. It wasn't even difficult at all, but I just wanted it to be finesse. We'd also do many other great tunes that year including a piece called "A Crazy Little Thing Called Love. "This was a great jazz tune and really my first introduction to swing music. I believe we also did Glen Miller's "In the Mood" that year. What a great year. It was also during that year that I would get introduced to jazz band at the high school level. They were so much more talented than our jazz band was, and I wanted to be just like them. Once again, I would become very fond of a girl that was in the jazz band. I would say that with girls, a common thing in my life has been to be attracted to an athletic female or a talented musician. Of course, I'm also attracted to the famous actresses. I would like to have a girlfriend so much.

Eighth grade would also be memorable for me as I'm sure it was for much of you. It was the 1999-2000 school year. I can recall that I wasn't quite sure what to think about this whole Y2K thing that was a big fuss. Now it's simply just a thing of the past that no one probably even remembers but at the time this was such a big deal. By the time December 31st, 1999 got here I had been convinced by the media that the world was going to end when the clock struck midnight. I was really interested in this but, yet I didn't think much of it. I was too busy escaping into imagination and having imaginary friends. I'm writing this in 2009 and obviously we're still here and the world's still breathing. We avoided a disaster.

My Introduction to IU and more importantly the "IU School of Music"

It was during my eighth-grade year that I was introduced to Indiana University in Bloomington, Indiana. I have to say that my band director, Mr. Flanagin was a huge IU fan. Of course, being alum of the university, he had reason to be a fan. He was crazy about IU basketball and football. At that time, he had a very good reason to boast when he came into school about his Hoosiers and the basketball team as Bobby Knight was still in command. That isn't exactly the case in 2009.

Contrasting Opinions

As it just so happened my father hated the Hoosiers. I think more importantly he strongly disliked Bobby Knight. So naturally growing up and being taught to hate the Hoosiers I wasn't a huge fan myself when I met Mr. Flanagin. In fact, if it wasn't for him I probably never would have had any interest in them or going to the university as a student. Now most of the extended family on my mom's side loved Bobby Knight and the Hoosiers. It would often be a little heated when they were discussed at a family gathering. I felt like I couldn't like the Hoosiers because my dad didn't want me to, so I just never said much about them myself.

Mr. Flanagin was probably the first person to really discover my talent for music and trombone. He talked to me a lot about going on and playing further. Possibly even majoring in some sort of music in college. He informed me that I would need to purchase an intermediate trombone to continue playing though as I was quickly out growing my beginning one. Getting a new trombone was the best thing I'd ever done as I think it improved my playing even more.

Mr. Flanagin talked a lot about the IU School of Music to me. As some of you very well may know the IU School of music is one of the best music schools in the country and world. There's Julliard and then IU. There are other universities in the states who'd like to argue this, but I haven't seen anyone that tops IU or Julliard.

I would become very interested in IU and a possible career in music. I would begin listening to more classical music compositions and practicing harder. In Eighth grade I had the opportunity to participate in an IBA or Indiana Bandmasters Association honor band. It was a great experience for me as they take you in for the weekend and you rehearse for a day with other students that you've never met before. The best part about being in an honor band was the fact that you have the best players from each school in the band. So, your weakest link is the best player from some school. Therefore, the playing level of the ensemble increases significantly. I enjoyed eighth grade band so much however the rest of the year outside of band was quite a struggle for me.

During both my seventh and eighth grade years I had the opportunity to play trombone in the school's talent show. We always had a few people from the jazz ensemble get together and play one of our favorite pieces. This was a lot of fun for me. I was kind of nervous about playing for the entire school though. At that time, it was one thing for me to play in front of adults but to perform music that wasn't necessarily considered to be popular by the student body was a little more embarrassing and challenging.

Moving On

Eighth grade had come and gone. Middle school seemed to blow by extremely fast. Overall, I'd say that middle school was fun, but also challenging both socially and academically. Now that middle school was finished I was moving onto high school. I'd spend four years of my life in high school and I would say that it was an interesting for years for me. From being bullied and picked on to being literally punched and pushed around. The next four years would be very harmful to my self-esteem and I'd say that they were also pretty life changing. I was going to be a very small fish in a very big sea and I'd find myself at the bottom of the totem pole once again.

7 FOLLOWING FRESHMAN

I believe that there are several advantages to having the diagnosis in the elementary years. One of the major ones is that the individual will grow up knowing that they have Asperser's Syndrome and be very aware of where they have difficulties, rather it be at school, play group, home, or anywhere where people may be around.

If someone is aware of having Asperser's or any form of Autism at that young of age they may be able to receive the right kind of help in school. I would recommend that if you have a child who's been diagnosed that you report this to the school. Also report this to the child's individual teacher as he or she will be better able to assist your child.

There are several good things about reporting this to the school. Once the school is aware that the child has a disability there are several things that they can do to aid. They may already have special education teachers on staff and if they don't they will begin the search to find someone to help your child. Some schools even go as far as to hire someone who is educated in Autism and can provide adequate assistance to make sure the student is successful in his or her academic endeavors.

A lady that has been a tremendous help to me is a perfect example of how the school corporation may and should try and assist you. Kara Skaggs is now a behavioral consultant and works with people with disabilities. Kara has a bachelor's degree in special education from Purdue University, in West Lafayette, Indiana.

When Kara first graduated with her bachelors she accepted a special education position with Fort Wayne Community Schools. She was put into a high school situation where she would spend six hours a day with these special education students. She quickly found that there were about eight kids who had autism.

I think currently Fort Wayne Community Schools was probably a little uneducated in the autism field and they weren't sure as of exactly how to handle the situation. Also, I would suggest that this was probably at a time where we were gaining more knowledge of autism and becoming more educated in giving a diagnosis to someone. So, because of that this could have very well been the first time that Fort Wayne Community Schools would see such a high number of autistic students in their corporation.

What happened after band camp? The first day at a new school and much more.

The conclusion of band camp meant that the summer had come to an end and it was time for students to put their thinking caps back on and head back to school. I remember it being late August of the year 2000. It was a hot summer day and I was headed into a new building with new teachers and many new students in which I had never seen before. I remember feeling completely overwhelmed about the new situation that was be presented to me. I remember feeling a little scared as I wasn't sure what I was getting into. I'd heard all the rumors about how seniors liked to come around and put freshman inside of a locker and lock them in or how they like to stuff freshman in the trash cans. I remember being totally aware of this and being extra careful about the first week or two of school. Whenever I was in the hallway I tried to be on the lookout for the "big" kids who were going to pick me up and harm me. I am happy to report that I never ended up being stuck in a locker or a trash can. What a huge sigh of relief.

There were so many people within the high school. I can tell you that I graduated in a class in which I was eventually able to know who almost everyone was. There were probably a handful of people that I can think of that I couldn't tell you what their name was to this day.

Huntington North High School had what they called a block four program. This program no longer exists at HNHS today. The day was divided into four ninety-minute periods with lunch added into the mix. First period was marching band. We would get to school at 7:50 in the mornings and then immediately must hit the marching field for rehearsal. This was a poorly designed schedule but Huntington County Community Schools. This would mean that in late August and early September when the temperature was still in the 80's and sometimes the 90's and very humid at times that students would have to be outside on the marching field for rehearsal and then must go inside and go about the rest of their day in the sweaty clothes that we inquired during first period. It would make a lot more sense to have marching band be the last period of the day which is the way it is at Huntington North today.

Marching band would provide many experiences for me. Experiences that kids just don't get to have if they aren't involved with an extracurricular activity. I believe that it's extremely beneficial for someone who's on the autism spectrum to become involved with extracurricular activities at the middle school and high school level. Maybe it's something that's a special interest to them. This is also a good way of attempting to make friends. For us on the spectrum that must work so hard at making friends, making them through a special interest can seem easy for us. I would also say that making friends through the special interest is a lot less stressful for the autistic individual.

Think about this. When an autistic individual is setting out for the sole purpose of trying to make friends and form a friendship they can become so focused on it that it is overwhelming to them. The person on the spectrum must work so hard to think through every social situation to the point that it can emotionally drain them. By making friends through a special interest, the autistic individual becomes more focused on the interest as opposed to making friends. While there's no guarantee that a friendship just going to randomly appear in one's lap as a gift, I believe that it's highly more likely that the individual on the spectrum will be able to talk to people in a more comfortable way which could allow the NT individual to become interested in them.

Again, knowing what I know now and thinking back to my past I can recall the situations where for whatever reasons I was more focused on doing something rather it be playing basketball or playing trombone than I was in making and developing friendships. It was these days to where I had some successful social interactions with individuals. Never to the point to where amazing friendships would blossom out of it but at least I was able to socialize. This happened because I wasn't aware of my diagnosis and wasn't focused on trying to fix me or change me.

Academics during freshman year

Academics became increasingly more challenging for me as I went through school. During my freshman year I can remember struggling more so than before. This was obviously due to the amount of change that was going on in my life. I can remember times to where I'd try to focus on a homework assignment and just not be able to focus on it for more than five to ten minutes at a time. I didn't really think too much of this at the time though. I just thought that this was how hard school was supposed to be. It wasn't until after I received my diagnosis and started studying up on Asperger's syndrome and autism that I began to realize that my problems with academics during high school were obviously due to having Asperger's Syndrome.

This is another situation in which being aware of having

Asperger's Syndrome would have been significantly beneficial to me. Had my parents or myself known of this like I do now I could have reached out for academic support from the school system. I honestly believe that I would have been an all A's and B's student if not an all A's student had I been able to get help and receive the proper support. Again, I can't stress how important it is for parents who notice their child starting to struggle in school to check into the possibility that your child may or may not have Asperger's or autism. There's no harm in checking. The results of finding out are tremendously important not only to your child during high school, but also in early adult hood as he or she may be put into some circumstances that they may not be able to handle without knowing they have a diagnosis and getting help.

Fall 2000 Marching Band Tour

High school marching band would be much more intense than I could ever imagine. In middle school I think it was still about the students learning how to get around the instrument as I like to call it. They spent more time rehearsing and preparing than they did performing. While we would still spend much more time rehearsing than we did performing, high school marching band provided anywhere from fifteen to twenty-five performances between the months of August through October. It was during this group of performances in my freshman year to where I would feel left out. I thought I was weird, and different than the other students. I would try so hard to connect with them and while they'd talk to me for a moment or two they would quickly move on to someone who I guess was much more appealing or interesting to them.

This is what I will refer to as the 97/3 equation. I've come up with this over the past few years after trying to become friends with different people. Basically, what I'm saying is due to the circumstances the person with an Asperger's or autistic diagnosis must put 97% of the effort into forming the friendship while the NT individual is only willing to put about 3 % into it. The NT individual will acknowledge a person on the spectrum if the person on the spectrum is trying desperately to get their attention and approval but will never give them much more than a moment or two of their time and become quickly uninterested. This is quite simply because they think that someone on the spectrum is different or weird. Society has a history of trying to avoid something that's different or weird.

The Bus Rides

High school marching band consists of going to perform at parades. It also consists of performing at the high school's football games as well as traveling to and performing at marching band contests throughout the state of Indiana. For me one of the most traumatizing experiences was the bus rides to and from the performance event.

I wanted to be "cool" and fit in with the other kids so much. However, for me that was just not something that would be possible. It's like there was something in me that was blocking me from being like the other kids that I so desperately wanted to become friends with. I remember getting onto the buses and seeing all the other kids sitting together and laughing and having a good time. I wanted to sit with someone so bad, but no one would want me to. Often, I'd sit in a seat by myself but whenever this wasn't possible I'd be forced to come out of my comfort zone and ask someone if I could sit with them. I remember feeling so bad for asking them or bothering them with a stupid question. Sometimes I would hear "no" and other times I'd here a "yes." With the yes answers it was almost like they said yes but with a look of discuss on their face.

For me the bus rides to and from performances wouldn't be a social event at all. Due to the lack of friendships and the fact that there would really be no one on the bus that wanted to talk to me I would quickly do some escaping into the imagination and imagine the marching show that was getting ready to take place. I visualized every step of the show from warm ups until we would get off the field. You might say that I'm an expert of the show because I spent so much time visualizing it. In fact, to this day I can still tell you almost every single note and move that I had to do in every single one of my marching shows in high school. I would go so far as to say that I could have even marched someone else spot in the show since I was so focused on it and visualized it so often.

I was often disturbed at the other kid's behavior on the buses. To me this would become a quiet time of preparing for the upcoming show. It seemed like for these other NT students the bus rides to and from the competitions and parades would become a social hour or game. There would be so much yelling and screaming, even throwing spit balls at one another that I would often feel as if I was at a zoo rather than sitting on a school bus with a bunch of high school kids.

Obviously, there's a significant difference between performing at the high school level to performing at a professional level. There's even a huge difference between the high school level and the college level. College and professional level musicians know that the time before the show is a time of focus and concentration. A time of thinking situations through and visualizing the performance. This would be something that I started doing as early as eighth grade. Unfortunately, in a high school setting not too many students are there for performing. They're more there for the socializing and having something to do with their time. As I will talk about a little later, high school marching band rehearsals were miserable for me due to this. While college and professional musicians are all about having a good time, they can realize and comprehend when it's appropriate to goof off and have fun as opposed to when it's not. The time for goofing off and having a good time comes after the performance has been completed. Before the performance is a time of intense focus and concentration. The best performing ensembles are not always the most talented musicians from a technical standpoint. However, the best ensembles are the ones that can flip the switch and get into the moment of the music and concentrate at such an intense level that nothing else can disrupt their thoughts.

Getting Teased

Throughout my high school career, I was constantly teased

for how I took things so seriously. Especially in the music world. I was so intense with performing and practicing my instrument and the other kids just couldn't comprehend why I would be so interested in practicing. I think to them practicing was a drag and something that they didn't want to do. For me practicing to this level would eventually pay off for me.

High school marching band would also be a time of physical abuse from the older students. I can remember often getting pushed around while standing in a group of people. I remember instances to where other boys would come up to me and do something that they called a "T" bag. This was extremely painful. I hated having this done to me but to fit in and be friends with these people I would try to cope with it and let them do it to me repeatedly. There were other times in my life in which I have been physically abused in some shape or form but because I was so desperate for friendship I kept staying around these people trying to gain their approval. All I wanted was a good friend or two to like me and not treat me so bad. I've known people who said they're my friends but did all kinds of this stuff to me. People that have tried to take money from me or tell me because they were a senior and I was a freshman it was my place to pay for their meals, movie tickets, or various other things. Due to a lack of education and not knowing and understanding that I had Asperger's syndrome (not even knowing what Asperger's I was would let this happen to me repeatedly. I didn't dare tell anyone because I didn't want to get anyone in trouble. There was a time to where people thought it was cool to randomly poke me in the face. This would be something that they'd do to other students as well, but I remember hating it and wishing that they'd stop. As some of you may or may not know people with Asperger's or a form of autism often have a comfort zone in which they can feel completely uncomfortable if it's breached. Well for me this would be breaching that comfort zone and it would hurt. I think back to these high school days now and wonder to myself, "How did I let this happen?" "Why did I put up with this for so long?" Unfortunately, I did because I wanted that acceptance to happen so badly. I really believed that for me to be accepted and liked by others that this was something that had to happen. This was normal and happened to every kid. I was unable to pull myself out of abusive relationships with people in which I would think were my friends because I valued having someone to hang out with so much that I couldn't pull away.

Importance of the individual being aware of what's going on.

Looking back at everything that's happened to me in my life, I've now set out on a mission to make sure that the same things don't happen to other children on the autism spectrum. I would hope that we would be able to recognize the signs of this happening in our schools and take steps to prevent them from occurring. Unfortunately, the person with an autistic diagnosis may be gullible and unable to even tell when this is happening. I mean sure they can tell when someone's hitting them, and it physically hurts, but often they have a very high tolerance for pain. The sad thing is that sometimes even if an autistic person can recognize that some form of abuse is going on that they don't often have the necessary skills of knowing how to report it. This leaves the person in a completely vulnerable and dangerous position.

Therefore, it's so important that our teachers are trained and able to recognize signs of autism in their students at early ages. We must become more aware of this so that we can prevent abuse from happening. To me this is one of the most important things that we could do.

Back to marching band, the end of the first season.

The marching band season would end with the band receiving a division II ready at the Indiana State School Music Association (ISSMA) regional competition in Carmel, Indiana. Today ISSMA has updated their scoring system and is no longer on a Division I, II, III scoring system but instead they've went to a Gold, Silver, and Bronze rating. I was devastated that we didn't get a division I and go on to state. I loved competing and wanted to win and be the best. I remember seeing some seniors who were also devastated and some who were even crying as their high school marching careers had end. However, many of the underclassmen would just act as if nothing had ever happened and continue about their day laughing and having a grand ole time socializing with one another. Sometimes I wish I could have been just like them but other times I like my more serious approach to life and music. It's something that I'm good at and can provide something interesting for an audience to listen to so why shouldn't I take it seriously? I should note that I understand that both approaches are appropriate at certain levels and I see nothing wrong with having a good time and enjoying one's self. It's not all about winning at all but more about performing your best.

High School brings a new opportunity "High School Dances"

December of 2000, a cold wintery night just before Christmas would bring about the first dance of a freshman's high school career. This was an exciting opportunity for everyone. I was so excited to go to the dance and was really looking forward to it in a huge way. I would quickly think about tuxedo's, flowers for the girl, where to take the girl for dinner, how to open every door for her, basically how to treat her like a queen. Unfortunately, I was getting ahead of myself and forgetting one very important piece of the equation. The "girl" herself.

Suddenly I was puzzled. I had taken care of the pre planning for everything. Even made dinner reservations to a nice restaurant. But I didn't have the girl lined up. For some reason I wasn't exactly good at talking to girls. To this day this is something I'm still struggling with. More details on this in a later chapter. But I knew who a lot of girls were and thought a handful of girls were beautiful. Okay so I think I thought I was having was more along the lines of "they're the most beautiful and amazing person I've ever seen in my life. I knew who they were, knew which was interested in but the problem was I didn't know how to talk to them. Unfortunately, to ask someone to go to a dance with you, one must be able to talk to them. I would have to be able to initiate conversation with them and be bold and brave enough to ask them to be my date for the dance. This would be something in which would require me stepping out of my comfort zone and taking one of the biggest risks I'd ever taken in my life. The question I had next wasn't for her it was for me. I would ask myself. Am I capable of doing this?

Answering my own question.

Unfortunately, I would end up answering my own questions. Except for I remember I didn't answer the question with just one answer. Hundreds of answers popped into my head. After spending a few days thinking through this and trying to decide if I can ask her to be my date to the dance so many negative thoughts come to mind. Some of them were, "I don't know what to say to her." "She's too pretty for me." I'm not brave enough." She's too good for me." "She doesn't like me." I'm not as cool as the other guys she knows." "I'm too stupid for her. "I'm worthless." Even "I'm too fat and ugly for her."

I think it's but the fact that all these thoughts would immediately start rolling through my head was enough to quickly scare me out of asking anyone to go to the dance that year. However, I was determined, and I would even pre order some flowers on the Thursday before the dance thinking I would come up with the courage to ask someone to be my date on that Friday with the dance being on Saturday. I never did end up asking a girl, so I guess I just bought myself some flowers.

Caution Danger for an autistic individual (Physical and

emotional abuse"

For an individual on the autism spectrum there can be many things that could present a danger from them. Depending on the severity of the autism the dangerous could range from not being socially aware and making social mistakes or going as far as doing something that's dangerous and could cause them to get hurt or worse. These individuals on the spectrum are simply just not aware of the many dangerous that there are in this world. I know for me this has been very much the case through my entire life. I would be easily taken advantage of and put into situations in which I didn't really want to nor have any interest in being in. Therefore, I think it's crucial that we are aware of this information and can hopefully come up with a way of preventing someone with high functioning autism or Asperger's syndrome from being put into harmful situations.

How can we help teach people on the spectrum of the dangerous they may encounter in life?

There are a few great programs out there to help with educating people on the spectrum about abuse. One of the more helpful ones that I've encountered as an adult on the spectrum is a program called "Bringing the Birds & Bees Down to Earth: Sexuality & Sexuality Education for Persons with Autism. This program is done by Lisa Mitchell, LCSW. Lisa has a very interesting presentation and she teaches at a level that people on the spectrum can understand and relate to. She's also very good at teaching at a level that support staff and professionals in a field can relate to. I would highly recommend that this program be a must see for not only people on the autism spectrum but also equally as important support staff and other professionals who are working within the autism field.

While this program is taught with an educational perspective, Lisa has also managed to make her presentation entertaining. You will not only find this presentation an educational tool, but also as an educational tool that you could possibly learn and incorporate some things into your teaching and working with autistic individuals. This presentation in which I've seen is put out by "Autism Speaks" It's time to listen. You can find more information about "Autism Speaks" and this presentation by visiting autismspeaks dot org.

We just must continue to be aware that individuals on the autism spectrum do not think in the same way that NT's do. NT's are always cautious and aware of the dangers things that are out there in the world. In fact, sometimes I wonder if girls don't come with this internal instinct that sends an alarm off to them when something is a little different or out of place. While this is a great thing for a woman to have. It's important to remember that just because something appears to be a little different, it doesn't automatically mean something's wrong with them. There may be an inside factor that is not visible in the person Therefore because of the internal instinct that NT's seem to have they are quickly turned off by the autistic world. This is quite simple just a miss interpretation. As I have so often been told by other people on the autism spectrum. They feel that no one understands them or that they are constantly miss understood. This is something that we all must come together and work on by providing adequate education. Both to the NT's and the autistics. It's all about compromise. The autism individual must try and learn the norms of society and become more aware of appropriate and inappropriate actions while the NT individual must become more in tune with autism and how it affects the individual. This is something that I call the 50/50 compromise. I am going to give you a more in depth look at the 50/50 compromise in a later chapter. This is something that I'm going to try and be an advocate at promoting both across the United States and across the world. I believe in all my heart that this is something that we can accomplish. I also know that in my heart, autistic individuals mean no harm to anyone. They simply just don't have the brain capacity with the normal social skill set that the NT individual has, and this causes them to seem awkward. Let's all work together and try and understand each other.

8 ON THE OUTSIDE LOOKING IN

After a freshman year full of both success in music and failure in peer relationships I retreated to my home for the summer and didn't really go out much. Until I received my first job at Ponderosa Steakhouse in Huntington, IN. I was 16 when I first started working there. I will talk a lot more about my first job experience in the chapter "Asperger's and Employment, how do we help?" Later in the book.

So, after spending the summer doing many of the same things that I had been doing such as creating a make-believe world of friends and escaping into imagination whenever possible I would go back to school to become a sophomore. My sophomore year would be exciting in the music area as it was my first full year of playing trombone in the Huntington North Varsity Singers. The varsity singers were an amazing group of talented singers, dancers, instrumentalist and stage crew.

I had originally auditioned to be in the Varsity Singers (our schools show choir in the spring of 2000. There were four trombone players auditioning for three spots. There were two juniors and one senior auditioning. It was an honor to be auditioning for such a talented group. I remember that I was extremely nervous on the night of auditions because I didn't know anyone there. I did manage to play a solo well and had some success with site reading the ballad that we had to play. Eventually the three trombonists were picked, and I wasn't one of them. I was kind of disappointed at first, but I knew that these other students were older than me and had more playing experience than I had.

After the auditions, I went on with my summer. As summer came to an end it was time to head back to school. It was another interesting marching season. It was the best marching season out of all four years of high school for me. We had the best scores of any year during that season.

I still didn't like the bus rides and I didn't like all the yelling and screaming that went on during the bus ride. I noticed that some things such as randomly loud noises like screaming or yelling were starting to bother me. Now it seemed strange to me since I was so used to being around music that this surprised me. To this day this still amazes me as I love loud music but the strangest noises kind of disturb my train of thought.

I can recall a day during my sophomore of high school. In fact, I can envision in quite clearly as I'm sure so many of you can as well. The day was September 11th, 2001. For me that day would start out just like any day. I would wake up and get around for school and then begin the day. I started out taking the graduation qualifying exam that morning just like the previous day. However, we all know just how quickly that day would take a tragic turn.

The events of September 11ᵗʰ changed a lot of things in this country. I remember feeling sad for all these people that were hurt or killed in the attack. This leads me to my next topic of discussion here. I believe that people with Asperger's syndrome and Autism have the capability of feeling compassionate about people and things more so than their NT counterparts. I believe that this is due to the fact of how much emotional pain that they've suffered in their life. All this rejection and being misunderstood. I mean for me, I can totally relate to someone who's having a rough time in life and struggling with issues. My heart went out to the people that were killed and injured that day as well as to the family members of those that were injured or killed.

I think for me it's easy to relate to someone who is suffering because I can remember when I've felt like that in the past. I can still remember the days in which I felt like giving up and throwing in the towel. It's extremely difficult for someone who doesn't experience depression to understand the amount of pressure and pain a person is going through. I used to often wonder why people would try and tell me that it wasn't that bad and it's going to be okay. I was so frustrated with them that it drove me nuts. "They just don't get it." I would think. Now looking back on it I can understand why they didn't get it. They had never experienced the feeling to the level of intensity that I was experiencing it at. They couldn't possibly relate to an experience in which they've never had. You see, everyone is different and unique. I'm sure there are many NT individual's experience depression and anxiety, what I'm not sure of is to what level and intensity that they experience it at. This is something I would be curious to see a study done on.

Being called into action!

I remember that on a day in January the HNHS choir director Mr. John Wenning called me into his office. I had auditioned to be in his show choir backup band just a few months prior to that but didn't make it since there were many upperclassmen auditioning and I at the time was just a freshman. Mr. Wenning called me in to his office and asked me if I wanted to be in the show choir band for competition season. I was stunned. Hearing the show choir perform in middle school was exciting to me. It was that Broadway type style that I loved so much. Of course, I accepted his offer and immediately began practicing with the backup band to prepare the show. Joining show choir backup band was the best musical experience that I had in high school. This group was extremely talented and motivated. The Varsity Singers had a great leader who knew how to compete and win. He is one of those music directors that in my words, "just gets it."

While the performing aspect of show choir was extremely fun and entertaining for me, the social part of it would prove to be yet another nightmare for me. Once again, I was just a worthless tag along. At times it felt as if the other kids didn't even know that I existed or that I was there. When I was included again it led to be made fun of while playing a card game or being asked to get them something or do something for them. It was never about just being friends. For me I was looking for friendship and so desperately wanted and needed to be friends with these kids. Often when we'd sit in the bleachers at events I would feel out of place as if I didn't belong. While I was having all these feelings on the inside I never addressed them with anyone because in my mind they already thought I was weird and hated me so if I told them this then what would they think? They'd probably think that I was a creepy psycho. I knew I couldn't tell anyone and I also thought that these were completely normal feelings that I was having.

Celebrating a championship

One of the perks to be a part of such a talented group of musicians was the fact that we would often win grand champion at numerous show choir competitions in the state of Indiana as well as some in the surrounding mid-west states. I can remember the first time that the choir won the grand championship at a competition with me being a part of the group. People ran the stage and I thought that there was a rock concert going on. I was amazed at the level of celebration that was going on. This group was a much more dedicated group as far as work ethic than any other group that I'd ever been a part of. If I would have had the proper social skill set I think I really would have enjoyed this group.

The Varsity Singers would never finish a competition lower than fourth place when I was in the group and we would go on to win 11-15 competitions in my four years there. It was a huge success that led to many different opportunities. We had the opportunity to travel on two trips and perform on one. In the spring of 2002 we went to New York City where we had a chance to visit the world trade center site. What a somber moment. In 2004 we had the chance to take our show on the road and perform in Disney's Universal Studios in Orlando, Florida. These two trips were once again good experiences as far as the trip itself, but I would feel left out. It didn't help that I was unable to stay in a room with the other kids since I'd still had a bed wetting issue at night.

The hugging or should I say lack of hugging that lead to tears

As all members of the choir would quickly gather on the stage to begin celebrating being named grand champions of a competition people would start hugging each other. I like hugs and to me this would be an exciting thing. I can remember thinking to myself, awesome their hugging and then I waited, and I waited, and I waited some more, and then I waited some more. It was very rare that I would get a hug. The girls would run around hugging other guys like there was nothing to it and then it seemed like when they got to me they gave me the look of "oh gross, you're creepy, go away."

I was devastated. This would happen to me repeatedly at every show choir competition we would go to. "What was wrong with me I thought?" I couldn't understand why these girls would just avoid hugging me. "They must hate me." Or "I must be a completely fat, ugly, worthless, piece of trash I remember thinking to myself." I couldn't help from having these horrible thoughts about myself. I thought that I was a good person and I couldn't understand why it was so hard for me to make friends or why girls thought of me in such a negative why. I couldn't figure out what I had done wrong or what I did to them that would make them treat me this way? At times, I would often think that they hated me just for being born into the world. I didn't get it. Something was wrong with me and I had no clue what it was or how to fix it.

Walking into competitions from the bus.

When the bus arrived at a competition site everyone would get off the bus and line up to go inside the school. The Varsity Singers had a tradition of walking into a competition site together in couples. So, everyone went inside holding a guy or girls hand. For me this would have been amazing as for me to this day just holding a girl's hand would feel like I was on top of the world. However, I remember holding a girl's hand as I went into competitions twice out of more than fifteen competitions. For some reason I was always the one that would get passed over. I didn't have a clue why.

The comment that would not only change my major but change my life for worse.

I remember sitting in band one year with my fellow trombone players. There were a few kids in band and it was always a competition to see who the section leader would be. I was always the section leader in every ensemble (except when there were upperclassmen who were older than I am playing in the ensemble. It was one wintery day in 2002 and I was sitting in my high school band class. I was always a student who would spend countless hours upon hours in the practice room playing trombone. The other kids would always make fun of me and tease me because I had no life and practiced all the time. To me the frustrating part is that these kids would often be the same kids who would shun me and not even give me a chance to be their friend and hangout with them.

Well on this one day, the comment that one of the students made was more hurtful and emotionally damaging than any other comment anyone had ever said to me up until that point. I was sitting in my chair waiting to play my trombone when I heard the words "You practice your trombone so much that you're going to end up marrying your trombone and you'll never have a girlfriend." Now obviously most kids in a normal mind set with any sort of a good self-esteem about themselves would have just let a comment like that go in one ear and right out the other year. But imagine if you were someone who'd been laughed at, made fun of, pushed around, taken advantage of, and rejected all your life. You'd probably really analyze what the other kid said. I know that's what I did.

I remember being completely stunned that he'd said that. My jaw dropped to the floor. Immediately I would start over analyzing it and become obsessed just with his comment. This really hurt me and would influence some things that would happen later in my life. Was I wrong for practicing trombone so much? Was that why no one liked me?

I would spend the rest of that year being really lost. I wasn't sure if I belonged here. I would continue to try to develop peer relationships and for some reason it just wasn't happening for me. I quickly became more and more frustrated. It's important to note that all throughout my life as time went on and I became more aware that I had a problem; I kept trying harder and harder to find out what the problem is. It's really depressing to be able to recognize that you have a problem but not have the slightest clue as to what your problem is.

Working at Ponderosa would start to present many more problems. I thought maybe being at work would give me a chance to really fit in and feel like I belonged somewhere. Unfortunately, that didn't quite happen at all. I would quickly be pegged as someone who could be taken advantage of by people. The frustrating and sad part is that people who have autism or Asperger's syndrome simply aren't socially aware enough to recognize when someone's taking advantage of them or using them. We don't have the capability of recognizing this sometimes. Although sometimes I would be able to recognize it but because you really want that friendship to develop with someone you tend to stay in a bad situation. Let's make a comparison here for the NT world.

If I had a dime for every time in my life I've heard a woman say, "Well he treats me so bad, but I can't leave him." Sounds like an oxymoron. This is a very true statement though. What happens is that these women are tricked into falling in love with these men and once they're in love it's hard to leave no matter how bad she wants to. This would be the same situation to an extent. For example, I could often tell that someone was using me for money or using me to provide something for them but because I so desperately wanted friendships I stayed and didn't run. This is the biggest mistake and the costliest mistake I have ever made in my life. You see, staying there may make you feel good for a short period of time because that person is giving you some attention. But at the end of the day when you part ways you go home, and you realize that person doesn't care about you one little bit. They just wanted your money or something of value to them that you had. This is really damaging to one's self esteem.

Having someone to watch out for you.

Obviously as we know it's extremely difficult for a person with an autistic disorder to make friends. Therefore, this next thing is a difficult task, but I believe it's crucial for the person with Asperger's or autism to have someone to "look out" for them. Someone who's educated about the autism spectrum and understands that these individuals may not always be aware of making the right decision when it comes to being taken advantage of. It's more than likely that they will allow themselves to be taken advantage of even if they do recognize that it's going on. If we could just get one peer to understand our people, then we'd be taking a huge step toward success. It's extremely important that children in middle schools and high schools get education on autism. All students should receive some type of training and education. I would even go as far as saying that this is something we could start doing with them as early as fourth grade.

I know of a gentleman who does autism presentations for the local school corporations around here. He says that it's a huge hit and success with most of the students. I think it's great when I see people from the community reaching out and getting involved in educating people about autism and its effects on society. How else would these kids learn? It must come from someone who's familiar with it and someone who experiences first hand.

I think our teachers are great around here but teaching autism awareness is just something that they're not trained to do. The last time I checked there was no autism education class required for completion of a bachelor's degree in elementary education or secondary education. I realize that universities require that their students take a special education class or two, but this is simply not enough.

What I would like to see!

I would really like to see the schools hire someone who's trained in the field of autism to keep on staff always. I know that some schools have explored this idea but let's face it. The problem is simply in the budget. A school corporation in Fort Wayne, Indiana just had to eliminate nearly 100 teaching positions for the 2009-10 academic school year. In 2008-2009 the classroom sizes seemed a little big even to me but with eliminating 100 positions this is going to be a tragic thing. We're telling our kids that we don't value education enough to keep a teacher on staff to educate them? We are sending the wrong message.

While this corporation is planning on hiring some of these teachers back before the 09-10 school year starts next fall, they probably will not be able to hire all of them back. Since the Indiana Senate and House of Representatives have not passed a budget for 2010 these teachers are being let go and left hanging. What kind of message is this sending to the teaching profession in itself?

Finishing Sophomore Year

As the spring of 2002 came along I would continue to go to school and pray that I could fit in. I would pray that I would make friends and be able to have a normal life. I was able to recover somewhat from the comment the student made about my trombone practicing and resume playing trombone and practice. In fact, I would say that I probably practiced more than ever be for. I would have the chance to join the Fort Wayne Youth Symphony and begin taking private lessons from the principal trombonist of the Fort Wayne Philharmonic.

I would travel to Fort Wayne after school, on most nights after a music rehearsal to take a lesson from Mr. David Cook. David has an amazing teaching style that's not comparable to anyone else I know. It's a little different and it really motivated me to practice achieving my best. That year I would begin taking solo's to ISSMA competitions and receive superior ratings. I even went on to state. I had a new sense of motivation for music and was losing interest in the social world again. Once again, it seemed like I just wanted to create my little bubble and hide in it. It's so much easier to just create a make believe social life than to try and fit in to the real-world socializing. It's also a lot less painful.

My first real crush.

During my sophomore year I was in a German class with an amazing girl. We will call her Jennifer. She was also a member of Varsity Singers. After kind of getting to know her in German class I was very interested in her. Not only was she pretty but she was understanding and had an awesome personality. She made a great friend. In February of 2002, I decided that I liked her, and I was going to be brave enough to ask her out. Unfortunately, due to my lack of social knowledge I would not know how to go about doing this.

My approach was to go out and get her a necklace and a few other things in which I would proceed to give her after school and before a varsity singer's rehearsal on Valentine's Day. Somehow, she found out about my intentions though and tried to avoid me. As it ended up I was able to give her the necklace and other gifts except for now I felt bad because I knew that she thought that I was creepy.

However, to this day, I can still recall giving the gift to her by the lockers and having her say "You're a sweetheart" and then giving me a hug. You might be wondering why this was such a big deal to me. Well for a guy who'd never had much success around girls just to get a girl to say hi and talk with me was an accomplishment but getting my first hug from a girl was an amazing feat for me. It was something that I've always remembered, and I will cherish it for the rest of my life.

I can honestly sit here and say that the experience with Valentine's Day and Jennifer was the only real positive social experience that I can take away from high school. There were many other attempts at social success, but most would lead to failure, ridicule, and rejection.

Infatuation with a local television Celebrity

During my late freshman year of high school and into the beginning of my sophomore year, I started watching the morning news every morning when I woke up as I was getting around for school. It was during this time that Wane-TV News Channel 15 in Fort Wayne, Indiana had an excellent and award-winning morning newscast.

Tara Brantley and at the time Mark Mellinger (who has now been promoted to the evening news with Heather Herron) were the anchors on the morning show. I've always thoroughly liked both Tara and Mark as I think they really have a passion for reporting the news and are real down to earth people.

However, it was during this time around my sophomore year in 2001-2002 when News Channel 15 decided to bring on board another morning reporter to do some special reporting for the show. This reporter went around the city doing specialized reports during every morning show.

Her name was Nicole Minsky. She was so pretty and fresh out of college. I remember how when I would see her on the news I would just practically fall in love on instant. She did several reports throughout a one to two year stand I think. Her stay here was short lived because she was so talented and would eventually move onto bigger cities.

Nicole did anything from reporting from local restaurants in the mornings to reporting on snowfall out live in the snow. One of her stories included a visit to the hospital in which she had to get blood drawn for medical awareness week that was going on in Fort Wayne.

I became infatuated with Nicole and she was someone that I could look up to and she was also very pretty. I remember looking forward to the morning new show all the time. When I couldn't watch it, I would make sure I taped it and watched it later. It's so hard to explain this to neurotypicals in a way that they can understand but due to the amount of rejection that you receive as someone on the spectrum daily, you start to form these fake friendships with people you see on television. However, to myself, they didn't seem fake because they were the only friendships I was having. It was like as close to reality as it could get for me.

Nicole left Wane-TV News channel 15 in April of 2004. At that time, I was a little devastated that my favorite morning show person was leaving, and I'd no longer get to have a best friend in Fort Wayne anymore. Yes, for me, even when it's just a friendship that's been developed on television it still hurts when you no longer get to see them repeatedly. With the news reporters it almost seems as if it was even more real than the friendships with like movie stars and professional athletes that I'd created in my make-believe world.

It's more real because with like Nicole, she was a local reporter within the same city in which I was going to school and living. I saw her on the news five days per week and at that time I'd dreamed of growing up and marrying her. Obviously, I'm able to be a little more realistic in that aspect today as I'm a little older, but I'd still have to say that she's one of the coolest and sweetest girls that I knew in high school.

I've never actually met Nicole in person, but I'd always wanted to. To this day I'd still love to meet the people that I knew on television and created as make-believe friends for me. To this day, Cameron Diaz, Lisa Winter, and Nicole Manske are pretty much my three closest friendships that I've ever had. Now, I've never met Nicole or Cameron, I have seen Lisa in person playing basketball at Huntington North High School and I did get her autograph once, but I've never said anything more than hi to her. I would be tickled if I could just meet and have a little five to ten-minute conversation with either of these girls.

I remember that after Nicole left I felt a little lost because there wasn't that person to wake up to and listen to her talk every morning anymore. It was like losing a best friend. At the time I had no idea where she went. I didn't think about trying to find out where she had accepted a position at or anything like that.

After doing a little research in preparing me to share my stories in this book I found out that Nicole didn't go too far away from Fort Wayne. At least for then, she ended up down in Indianapolis, IN where she would work for Wish-TV. She covered racing both the Indianapolis 500 and the Grand Prix race in Indy. She also covered the Indianapolis Colts and Indianapolis Pacers. I also learned that Nicole is a huge fan of my all-time favorite football team, the Green Bay Packers.

Nicole stayed in Indy for about two years before accepting a position with the Speed Channel. She too that position in late May of 2006 and there she is a co-host for a talk show called "The Speed Report." It wasn't until recently that I've found this out so now I'm trying to figure out if I get the Speed Network on my television.

Nicole was a tremendous influence on me and someone that would pull me through every day by motivating me. It's so strange how someone who you've never met in person can be such an influence and great friend but again; I believe that it's due to the lack of capability in developing real friendships in real life that allows for this to happen.

People like Nicole may very well never realize how big of an influence they can play in someone's life because it's hard to get in contact with them to tell them thank you. But if Nicole, Cameron, or Lisa were ever to read this text, I would want to say "Thank you" to all three of them. They've helped me through difficult times without even knowing it and they've really been there as someone to talk to even if they couldn't hear me talking back. Once again, I'm not sure that I would be here today without having this make-believe world created in which I could create friendships with people. Thank you, Nicole, Lisa, and Cameron.

.

9 A DREAM DISCOVERED

The summer in 2002 would be spent working at Ponderosa Steakhouse and practicing my trombone. I would join and participate in a local summer concert band here in town. The remaining time was spent swimming at a pond my grandparents owned. Again, there was no real social interaction with peers other than the forced ones that would happen at work.

As I was beginning to get older and maturing quite a bit I was starting to become more aware of the situation that was going on. I was starting to become in tune with the fact that I really struggled socially. I couldn't figure it out but then at this point and time there was never really much desire to even attempt to figure it out. It was until later in my life that I would set out upon a remarkable journey to try and uncover the secret to my problem.

My job at Ponderosa would continue to cause me problems socially as I'd continue to be taken advantage of by both girls and guys that worked there with me. I'm not sure what it was but I just felt like I was a target or something. What was I doing that was so wrong that was causing me to be treated in this way?

The previous year while working at Ponderosa I was a cashier, and this was hard for me. No, not the mathematical part of the job, but more so the social part. I just didn't know what to say to the people as they went through my line. I had a hard time looking them in the eye. I was very anxiously nervous because I didn't want to say the wrong thing at the wrong time. I began to dread going to work to do that job, so I was relieved when they called me in and told me that they were moving me to a different position. I was now going to work with the food bars. There would be less socializing with customers and more time spent doing things that I sort of knew how to do and was somewhat good at.

This job was a little easier and less stressful for me, but I still struggled with my coworkers. I just wanted to be like them. I'd notice how a lot of times people would be whispering to each other and I often wondered if they were talking about me. This would not only happen at work but at school and pretty much any other social setting that I would be a part of. I became frustrated but at the same time Ponderosa would be become a security blanket for me.

Hanging out at Ponderosa

Even though I would get taken advantage and made fun of at work there were still some people I worked with at Ponderosa who would be nice to me and make me feel like I was someone of worth. While I never would develop what I would say a true everlasting friendship with any of these individuals it did provide a comfortable setting for me.

I found myself constantly hanging out at Ponderosa sitting there eating or just talking to people. This would become a security blanket for me as I didn't have a social life of my own. The only socializing that I was able to do is where it was pre planned or in a place to where it was just naturally designed to happen for me.

I would quickly become attracted to a girl in which I worked with and she really would make me feel good at least at work. It was just nice talking to her as I felt like this girl had at least a hart and was willing to listen. Unfortunately, my attempts to develop this friendship outside of work failed miserably and led to ridicule from her and others. I wasn't sure what I'd done wrong and once again I'd just assume that she along with everyone else hated me. This was extremely difficult me to deal with and I'd just try and become more withdrawn from society. Basically, only interacting with other people when I was forced to.

I withdrew to the make-believe world whenever I wasn't working. I would spend my hours at home watching movies that I'd recorded a few years back and imagining me having a much more successful social life. I would spend my days watching movies or playing trombone.

IU School of Music Interest

It was during that summer and the 02-03 school year that

I'd really become interested in pursuing a music education degree from Indiana University in Bloomington, Indiana. I began to explore the possibilities of auditioning for the IU School of Music and quickly start playing harder music. Mr. David Cook would prove to be a tremendous help for me in this area as well as Mr. Scott Hippest who was an IU alum.

I began to practice countless hours upon hours. I went to all region bands to play with some of the greatest musicians from across the state. I continued to try and keep up on my studies at school and kept playing in all the school ensembles. Between trying to go to school, working, and participating in musical ensemble rehearsals, I was so busy that I managed to be able to forget about most of my problems for at least a year or two.

My junior year is what I would say the best year of my high school career. I didn't try too hard to develop friendships because I was so busy doing the things that I loved to do and working. I enjoyed my job at Ponderosa. I would have liked it a lot more if I would have been able to fit in and avoid being tortured by being taken advantage of and even at times being physically tortured and abused. I never saw a reason as to why most guys had to be so tough and macho.

During my junior year I was able to make a trip down to Indiana University in Bloomington. I went down there on a Saturday and would spend the night and come home on Sunday. This was a good experience for me and I really enjoyed the university. It was a huge place and there were so many people there that I'd never seen before. I remember crowding into a dorm room with a room full of people for the evening. IU had a bowling alley on campus and we were all able to go bowling and bowling is something I enjoy. I used to be on a bowling league and was pretty good way back in the day.

Becoming more interested in girls!

As I continued to get older I noticed that girls became more and more attractive. I really wanted to be able to get a girlfriend, but I just didn't have any idea how to. Dances at school would come and go and I didn't have a date. I thought that there was something severely wrong with me. I couldn't understand why girls wouldn't give me the same chance that they were giving other guys. Luckily that year I was able to keep myself focused on the work at hand with school and with my musical talents. The junior year would come and go without too much trouble. I would start working forty some plus hours a week at Ponderosa between my junior and senior year and I'd become one of the best employees. This was also something that I could feel proud about. At that time, I was able to keep focused enough to at least perform my job to the best of my ability. I loved to be at work as it provided something for me to do with people around. I think at that point I was still trying to find myself. I was trying to find a group or a couple of groups who would just accept me and allow me to be their friends. The group that would accept me the best out of any of my life would be the people I worked with at Ponderosa Steakhouse.

My junior year of marching band would prove to be a horrible season. For some reason we had a horribly difficult show and probably the least talented marching band of all four years. I would get frustrated with that season as to me it would just seem like other students didn't care how good we were and how we looked to the public. I was at a performing level to where I just wanted to be the best of the best in the musical world. I needed to be able to be involved with a group of people who would be as highly motivated as I was to be as successful as possible.

I would get this opportunity when I played with the Fort Wayne Youth Symphony. Playing with the youth symphony was fun because it was mostly playing with very little talking. The students in the group were much more focused on making professional level sounding music than they were on having a good time. This was a great experience that I learned a lot from and would help me to become a better orchestra musician.

The friendship/acquaintance ratio

At this point in time in my junior year I had no idea about the friendship/acquaintance ratio. I didn't know what it was or that it even existed. It's something I came up with about three or four years ago that I've used as a way of explaining my social interactions with people. As I've stated multiple times in this book, I often tried extremely hard to develop peer relationships and make friends. I tried so hard that it came to the point in which it would become mentally exhausting. It seemed like the harder I would try and develop a relationship or friendship with a person the more that person would hate me or think I was creepy or psycho.

The friendship acquaintance ratio is a relationship between an autistic individual and a Neurotypical or NT individual. The autistic individual may have anything from autism to high functioning Asperger's syndrome. What happens is that the person with autism or Asperger's is trying so hard to develop a friendship with the NT. To the individual on the spectrum as soon as an NT individual so much as says "hi" to them and or smiles at them the NT has become the person's best friend. While the NT individual was just saying hi to be friendly and may not even be interested in learning the person on the spectrum's name.

You see Neurotypical individuals have established a social network that is full of many different people. It's full of many different types of friends. They have guys that are friends and girls that are friends. Some of them will even have a boyfriend or girlfriend. To the neurotypical individual meeting the person who's on the spectrum won't mean anything at all to them. Because they know how to develop friendships appropriately they know that you do not just make a friend from saying hi to them or by even smiling at them. The person with the autistic diagnosis doesn't understand this and even if he or she did, they still would have a hard time with it because it just makes them feel so good that they didn't get ignored or even worse.

So, what happens is that the NT person becomes the person on the spectrums best friend instantly while to the NT individual the person on the spectrum just becomes an acquaintance (someone they may or may not have an interest of seeing again. Due to the excitement in the person on the spectrum they will become overly anxious and want to develop a friendship with the NT individual quicker than the NT is comfortable with. This will cause then NT to accuse or assume that the individual on the spectrum is being disrespectful and purposely missing these cues or "common knowledge" about building a friendship that NT's come preprogrammed with. The person on the spectrum may end up calling the NT too much or too often or texting and emailing them too much. This can become overbearing to the NT individual and they will retreat and try and get rid of the individual on the spectrum.

I know that this is something that has happened to me time and time again. When you end up getting rejected or made fun of you can't understand because you just don't realize or comprehend what you've done wrong. For me even when someone would explain it to me it wouldn't make much sense and I just couldn't understand why they were reacting this way to me. I will talk much more about what I call the "texting game" in a later chapter.

As my junior year was ending I felt like I was treading water socially. My social relationships just weren't improving to the level in which I had wanted them to. Of course, I didn't understand nearly a tenth as much as I do now about autism and Asperger's syndrome. For the longest time once again, I just thought that people hated me, and it was a mistake that I was born into this world. Over the summer between my junior and senior year I would put even more time into practicing. I officially decided that I was going to audition to the IU school of Music in Bloomington, Indiana. I practiced a lot and repeated various technical exercises over and over until I had them down perfect. I would continue working close to forty hours a week that summer and I still struggled with some bullying at work. Again, I can't stress how important it is that we train autistic individuals and people who have Asperger's syndrome to report something when they have a problem with someone. No one else will be able to tell because Asperger's especially is such an invisible disability. If one does not tell or seek out help it could be harmful to not only his self-esteem but could end up being physically harmful. There were several situations in where guys would make verbal threats to me and tell me I was stupid, and I should do whatever they told me to. I was able to fight this off for a long time before I would give in to doing what a guy told to and when I did it was because I was convinced that I was stupid and didn't know anything and this guy knew it all. I would end up thinking that anyone but me was smart and that they had all the answers and I should listen to and do everything they told me to. This was a huge mistake and because I wasn't even aware of having Asperger's at this point I didn't think anything was wrong. I just thought that that was how people treated some people and I just had to accept it, deal with it, and move on. In fact, I think I feared reporting it to anyone because I wasn't sure if I would get threatened or hurt by the person I was telling on.

People with autism or Asperger's syndrome should become aware of who they can trust and who they can't. It's extremely helpful to let your place of employment know that the person has autism or Asperger's and get them involved. This will allow them to be on the lookout for any bullying that would be going on. They might even seek out a mature co-worker to explain the situation to and take the aspie or autistic individual in under their wing. This will help protect them. Please note that an autistic individual will work much better and faster if he or she is in a safe environment to where there is little or no threat of being hurt. I know for me my work has often suffered when I felt like I was in dangerous situations and I was stuck in them because I was working. One will become anxious and be less focused on the job and make more mistakes. Having a safety net or security blanket so to speak allows the individual to relax and focus more on his or her task. I truly believe that people with Asperger's are just as hard of workers as anyone else. They just must be put in an environment that is safe, with little or no distractions so that they can focus on their task.

Lack of awareness in an NT individual

To me it seemed like NT individuals often don't even realize when they are doing something to hurt an individual with an autism or Asperger's diagnosis. I really don't believe that most individuals intend on hurting someone. I believe that there are several things that they just don't know. I think they assume that every individual can look out for themselves and that they are willingly submitting to the request at hand. They may just think the person is being nice or that they are just someone who has a lot of money and is willing to throw it around. I feel that educating the NT world is equally as important as teaching and educating people on the spectrum about social skills. We must compromise and come to a mutual understanding of one another.

Danger Beware:

While I have just stated that I don't believe most individuals try and purposefully take advantage of, use, or hurt people on the spectrum, I do think it's important to be aware that there will often be at least one or two people in a crowd who will be able to tell that the person is incapable of standing up for themselves or saying no to someone. They will take advantage of this to the best of their ability. This has happened to me time and time again and because of the level of desperateness to have a friendship or even relationship with a girl I've kept putting myself in these situations, I've sometimes put myself into harm's way as well.

There is no good way to prevent ourselves to handle being put into a situation to where we are going to be taken advantage of, we must simply prepare ourselves and practice saying no to someone to avoid being used and hurt. We can do this by bullying education. We can teach people on the spectrum and yes even kids who aren't on the spectrum to detect a bully and try to stay away from them. We can teach them to be with someone always who knows that they are vulnerable and will try and protect them. Then of course we must teach them to know how to report any type of bullying or abuse that is going on.

Most school systems in the United States of America have

bowling prevention program in place at their schools. However, I've heard of instances to which the bullying program basically did no good. There was a case out of the state of Georgia somewhere to where a little boy ended up killing himself because the bullying was so bad at school. This wasn't a case of the student not knowing how to report it as he did report it to his mom and she reported to the school time and time again. The school simply denied the problem and aloud other students to continue bullying this kid. This concerns me because if they were bullying this kid to that extreme, then I have a hunch that they are probably bullying other students as well. Why do kids do this? To me it's completely illogical. It makes no sense at all to treat someone like that unless of course the person doing the bullying is hurting themselves and have no respect for themselves.

Being on the receiving end of so much bullying in my life I can't express to you the amount of pain that goes through the individual who is being bullied. It's like you're stuck inside of a horrible dream and trapped. No matter what you attempt to do you can never escape it. If you tell someone the bully will find out but if you don't tell someone he or she will keep bullying, you and could cause severe mental trauma. I hated going to school so often since I knew the class bully was going to be coming after me trying to do something to me in some way that could hurt me. I tried to avoid him most of the time. This was not always possible though.

Summing everything up before beginning a downhill spiral.

Let's briefly try and summarize the first seventeen or
eighteen years of my life in which I've shared with you so
far. Let me summarize some things that I think would be a
red flag and tell us we have a problem. It's important to
keep in mind that back in the early 1990's when I was in
elementary school that we simply just didn't know what we
know today, and we didn't have nearly as much of an
understanding as we do now. It wasn't until about 1996
when we first begun to acquire an understanding of the
CNS (Central Nervous System) and its effect on sensory
development. Therefore, in my case it wasn't easy to
recognize the sings of Asperger's Syndrome as we just
weren't aware of what we know now. Let me briefly
discuss what should be some red flags in my opinion that
may and should send off a single in a parent's head to say
"hey, I think we have a problem, let's go talk to someone
about it."

When I started school, I was held back a year due to a lack
of motor skills and trouble with simple tasks such as
writing or coloring. *Today this would tell me that I had
problems with sensory development as well as controlling
motor skills. Knowing what I know now I could
educationally tell myself that there is possibly a dis-
function in the CNS.*

I had problems with controlling ticks. I had a tick in my
head to where I would just randomly shake my head for no
reason. This was most likely do to Tourette's Syndrome.

*As we now know today, Tourette's can be a side effect of
having Asperger's syndrome or autism. I am not sure if we*

know why this is or exactly what about Asperger's causes this. Again, this is a big red flag.

Lack of ability to socialize with peer groups in early elementary years.

I was socially unaware of my surroundings and how to make and maintain friendships. With Eric, I got lucky as I think with being such a young age friendships kind of happen on their own and don't really need any facilitating to be successful friendships. As we get older it becomes more necessary to put some time and effort into the friendship and then also use some social skills to keep the friendship going.

Accidents with bed wetting and bowel movements.

I would often have problems with bed wetting and bowel movements. I recently read a study that said people with Asperger's syndrome could possibly have trouble with bed wetting as well as bowel movements. Again, this was a huge ah hah moment for me when I read that study about three or four months ago. Now I can finally make my mother understand that I wasn't doing it on purpose.

The development of special interest and then losing track of the real world and creating a make-believe world.

I now know that it's common for people with autism or Asperger's syndrome to develop a special interest or two. In doing this they will become experts in their special interest area and they may lose interest in other areas. Some may lose interest in socializing in general.

Again, as we've talked earlier in the book. Autistic individuals will often create their own make-believe world to escape the pain of the real world. I have done this time after time again hoping that my make-believe world would somehow become my real world. I've tried to change who I was in real life because I had imagined that I was someone else in the make-believe world. This can be and usually is extremely dangerous and harmful when it becomes too intense.

These are five very important indicators in which I now look back on in my life which tell me that I may have had a problem or that something just wasn't right. I sometimes wish that the knowledge that's available today could have been available to professionals and teachers back in the early 1990's when I was in school so that my Asperger's could have been detected and I could have worked hard to become as normal of an NT as possible. However, this isn't the case anymore as I know it's much too late for me to fix myself and become a perfect NT, and I wouldn't want to be a normal NT individual now either as I wouldn't really be who I am. I believe that this is who I'm supposed to be and I'm currently in the process of continuing to accept my diagnosis and not only live with it but use it to make the world a better place for everyone.

This is a transitioning point in the story of my life. You would think a normal transitioning point in someone's life would come after their senior year of high school, but for me I think my transition would begin towards the end of my junior year and into my senior year. While my senior year would prove to be a fun year as far as extracurricular activities for me, it would become more and more miserable as far as socializing goes. I would become more and more depressed and lost in who I was. The next part of this book is going to take you directly inside of my brain as I graduate high school and begin my college career.

Included in this part of the book you will find enclosed journal entries with dates on them. These are very personal things to me, but I feel that it's important to share with the world. This will let you directly inside the head of someone who's living and dealing with the side effects of having Asperger's syndrome. It is my hope that by reading these professionals and NT individuals can gain more understanding as to what goes on inside the brain of someone who is dealing with rejection, being bullied, taken advantage of, rejected, and ridiculed daily. (Please note that these journal entries will not be edited as I want them to appear the way that they were written. There will be some grammar and punctuation mistakes and some spelling errors. When someone is feeling these emotions taking care of grammar and spelling is the last thing that's on their mind. The only thing that's on their mind is getting these thoughts out of their head and onto paper so that they feel better. Also, names of individuals that appear in the journal entries have been changed to a different name to protect that person's identity. While these were real life interactions with other people I do not feel it would be right to reveal their real names. I hope that you will be able to use this and take something away from getting the thoughts from directly inside the head of a person with Asperger's Syndrome.

10 A CHAPTER CLOSES

It was finally here. Senior year. I was ready to move on with my life. I began the year with lots of excitement and high hopes of being successful both in the music world as well as in the social world. I would continue to try and develop peer relationships with other students and would again struggle in this area. As you may be noticing, struggling with peer relationships is something that would be a struggle for me repeatedly. It wouldn't be something that would just naturally go away on its own. There was a great reason for this, but I didn't know why that was at the time.

Marching band would start out with a high note as I had quickly learned that the band directors had decided on a show called "Kipawatissmo" for my senior year. In this show there were three movements and two of them were arranged to start with trombone solos. The middle movement or "ballad" had a baritone solo in the middle of it. It was very lyrical and smooth, so it would be something that would be much more difficult to play on a trombone. I really enjoyed the music to the show; I just wish we could have had a more talented group to perform it at times. Not so much a more talented group but a more determined and dedicated group that would be more interested in performing the music to the best of their ability. Again, I was a musician who even in high school, wanted to be a professional musician and perform at a professional level of play.

I would begin preparing for my Indiana University School of Music audition the previous summer. I would start preparing one of my all-time favorite trombone solos. A piece called "Concertino for Trombone" by David Ferdinando. This is probably one of the more challenging trombone solo's out there on the market. It's a very demanding piece technically but also a very demanding lyrical piece.

When I first heard a gentleman by the name of Christian Limburg playing this piece I quickly fell in love with it.

Christian Limburg is one of the more famous professional trombonists in the world. He's put out several recordings of trombone solo performances. He has one of the most lyrical trombone voices of anyone that I've heard play in my life. Christian Limburg's rendition of Concertino #4 would be an inspirational piece for me. It motivated me because I wanted to play it just as good as he did if not better. I was always motivated by playing with or competing with excellent trombonist.

Frustrations and almost dropping out of high school

marching band

It was the middle to end of September and I became really frustrated with the other kid's in marching band because they didn't seem to take being there seriously. As I've stated before, the previous three years bothered me, but this year would bother me more so than the others.

Eventually I would get to a point to where I wanted to just drop out and get out of there because it felt like a huge waste of time. I could be spending my time on my personal practice or even studying rather than having to waste five minutes every time the directors would ask the students to be quiet before we could start playing or marching. I managed to stick it out and put up with all the frustrations and finish out the season and I'm glad I did because I love marching band.

We would eventually make it through that marching season with a gold rating at the ISSMA District Contest and then receiving a Silver rating at the ISSMA Regional competition in October of 2003. I was disappointed with the result as it was always my dream to march on the RCA dome floor in Indianapolis, IN. Unfortunately, that dream never came true and now it has no chance of ever coming through because the stadium has been torn down and the Indianapolis Colts now play at Lucas Oil stadium.

I would begin preparing for my Indiana University School of Music audition the previous summer. I would start preparing one of my all-time favorite trombone solos. A piece called "Concertino for Trombone" by David Ferdinando. This is probably one of the more challenging trombone solo's out there on the market. It's a very demanding piece technically but also a very demanding lyrical piece.

When I first heard a gentleman by the name of Christian Limburg playing this piece I quickly fell in love with it. Christian Limburg is one of the more famous professional trombonists in the world. He's put out several recordings of trombone solo performances. He has one of the most lyrical trombone voices of anyone that I've heard play in my life. Christian Limburg's rendition of Concertino #4 would be an inspirational piece for me. It motivated me because I wanted to play it just as good as he did if not better. I was always motivated by playing with or competing with excellent trombonist.

I would take that piece to that state ISSMA Solo & Ensemble competition in late January of 2004. I would receive a perfect score at the contest both at district and at state. This was very commendable as most students don't receive perfect scores at the state level. I was proud of myself for achieving this feat and it motivated me even more for my audition that would be coming up just to weekends later.

This was a busy time of year for me as I was balancing all the solo & ensemble contest along with Varsity Singers show choir competitions and of course preparing for the biggest day of my life.

Meanwhile I was still balancing the work schedule back at Ponderosa. This was becoming more complicated as there was starting to be some trouble with the general manager at

Ponderosa. He was one of my favorite people there. However, somehow, he'd get himself into a messy situation and eventually get fired from the company. They brought in another manager who would eventually take his place. At first, I wasn't a fan of this manager and struggled with the transition.

I would say like most things in life for someone dealing with Asperger's or Autism changing out of a routine can be a very difficult thing to do. Therefore, when this new manager came in and had new ideas and new procedures I was a little confused as to how to react to them. The change seemed to go okay with only a few minor speed bumps, but I would say it was a struggle. I think maybe the other employees adapted to change much easier than I.

Meanwhile back at school I was having a hard time with some higher-level math classes and didn't really seem to be able to focus too much on homework or trying. I think with everything else going on homework was the last thing I had on my mind. I mean there was preparing for the IU audition, marching band, varsity singers, jazz band, and of course work. I was also trying to play in the Fort Wayne Youth Symphony at the time as well as taking private lessons from the principal trombonist of the Fort Wayne Philharmonic. I didn't really have much time for a social life therefore I think my senior year may have been a little easier on me as far as being depressed as I wouldn't allow myself time to get down in the dumps over my lack of ability of developing friendships with the other kids.

The Days Leading Up to the IU School of Music Audition

In the final days leading up to the Indiana University School of Music audition I would not only become very focused on the outcome and goal that I had in mind, but I'd also become very anxious about it. I had never had a problem with becoming anxious before playing in front of anyone in my life but for some reason this time it was different. Of course, this was the biggest performance I'd ever been a part of in my lifetime up to that point. I was playing a trombone solo in front of three very respected trombonists who are on faculty at Indiana University in Bloomington.

Professors Peter Elefison, Dee Stewart, and Carl Lente would all be listening to me and critiquing my playing. I was extremely nervous and excited all at the same time. Luckily for me I did so much ensemble playing while in high school that I didn't have to worry about being in shape or not. My chops were golden. Of course, if one's going to be auditioning to the IU School of Music they had better not have to worry about their chops not being ready for the performance.

In the final days I was extremely busy as it was getting close to Varsity Singer's competition season. This was an intense time for the show choir as during the final week of preparation for competition season we would often have rehearsals every night. It was our last chance to polish up the show before we took it out on the road to compete with other schools.

I remember in the final week heading into the competition season I had a scheduling conflict. I probably tended to get myself involved in too many ensembles as I would often have conflicts and must pick and choose which ones I should attend. This was obviously creating a huge organization problem that I didn't like dealing with. As those of you on the spectrum know keeping things organized can be a difficult task for us. For some reason or the other we just aren't too good at balancing things.

So that February evening where I had a conflict was a night in which the Varsity Singers had an evening rehearsal scheduled from 6pm-9pm. Meanwhile, the Fort Wayne Youth Symphony also had an evening rehearsal scheduled from 5:15pm-7:45pm. With Fort Wayne being about forty-five minutes away from Huntington, where I lived this would make for an interesting controversy. Somehow, I had to be in two places at one time. Well I ended up splitting the time. I would go to the Fort Wayne Youth Symphony rehearsal but leave at 6:15pm. Then I jumped on the freeway and drove about eighty or ninety miles per hour to get back to Huntington North High School on time to rehearse with the Varsity Singers. Without even having time to eat or relax in between, I would get out my instrument and be ready to play the show choir show.

That evening we had a guest clinician who would often come in and work with the choir and backup band. They had run the show once without me being there and I remember as I was walking in the clinician accused the band of not being loud enough. Well, I was someone that was often known for my ability to play loud. Let's just say, I have a good set of lungs on me and I can push amazing amounts of air through the horn. Well when I get there, and we ran through the show a second time, all the sudden he said that the band was too loud. This was usually a good thing to hear although I'll admit there can be times when playing too loud is not necessarily appropriate.

For someone who didn't have very much success in anything other than music in his life, just getting any kind of a compliment at all would make me put a beaming smile on my face. Even if it was at something that I already knew I was good at I would still like it when someone would take notice and compliment me for a job well done. This was something that I think was able to help get me through high school. Without this I just wouldn't have had anything successful going on in my life. You might say that I used music as a tool of making myself not only feel better but as a sense of acceptance. I was accepted by others through my music and not for my socializing.

The Audition

For some reason I had ended up being scheduled to work on the night before my Indiana University School of Music audition. This wasn't such a good thing as I would have to spend the night before the audition working and trying to interact with other employees and customers. This was generally a very stressful task for me and it would demand all the attention and effort that I had. With the audition being the next day my attention was supposed to be more so on that but because of having to work I was kind of "scatter brained and roaming back and forth between thinking about work and the audition itself.

The night before I was supposed to audition at Indiana

University we had a horrible ice storm. The roads got bad and I remember being hesitant as if I even wanted to go the next morning to audition. I was supposed to be down in Bloomington by 8:00AM that morning and to be there on time that meant leaving between 4:00-5:00AM. I remember hesitating all night long at work thinking that we shouldn't go because of the weather. But now looking back on it I think I was more scared of afraid of auditioning than I was worried about the weather.

I had never had any problems playing my trombone in front of anyone and I was just naturally in the zone whenever I played. But this time do to the magnitude and meaning of the performance I was a nervous wreck.

My parents were able to calm me down enough to get in the car and head down there for the audition. I remember the drive quite clearly. It was snowy and icy. The roads were a mess and we had to drive really slow which would drive me even more crazy as it would give me more time to think and over analyze the days ahead.

When I got to Bloomington I was amazed at the site. There were so many people there on campus and I immediately heard students warming up and practicing in the practice rooms. For those of you who have never been to Indiana University in Bloomington, Indiana, I think it's one of the college campuses worldwide that is a must visit. You must see this university in the fall and spring as it is gorgeous.

The first day I was there I would spend most of the day filling out paper work, talking to people who were affiliated with the school of music and taking test. Yes, I said test.

This was not your standard university testing either. This was IU. One of the best music schools in the world. These tests would determine what level of theory and piano you would be in should you end up being one of the lucky ones to be chosen and accepted to the school of music. This was a very rare thing though as there were always so many kids auditioning that being one that would be selected is like a once and a life time thing. Let's just say it would be a tremendous musical accomplishment to be accepted to such a prestigious university.

I remember being very anxious as I was taking the theory test. I was generally very good with anything to do with music, however at our high school there wasn't much of a theory program as is the case at most high schools. Once entering college as music major, you spend more time working on and learning music theory and ear training. So, you'd think that with more time being spent learning theory and ear training that one would expect to spend less time practicing and rehearsing right? Wrong, in fact, if anything the amount of time spent practicing and rehearsing should increase significantly.

Being so anxious about the theory test I think was due to having Asperger's Syndrome. I of course wouldn't have any idea at the time as to why I was so extremely nervous. Looking back on it now that solution makes perfectly good sense. Playing wasn't so much of a problem but the test was nerve wrecking. This leads me to my next point.

Moment of Truth

The day was Saturday, February 7th, 2004. It was finally

here. Today I would experience my moment of truth. It was time to see if all the days, weeks, months, and years of practice had finally paid off. Was I going to be able to complete a huge step in the process of making my dream of becoming a professional trombonist come true. The time was now. Not later.

After seeing three other students from my high school audition for the IU School of music in each of the previous three years before me and not getting in, I was extremely nervous and afraid that I wasn't going to get in either. However, deep down in my heart, I knew that I was good enough. There was something about me and my determination of becoming the best that would push me and pull me through.

That morning I woke up early and left the hotel with my day to head over to the school of music building where the auditions were taking place. Each instrument was stashed off in their own little private section of the building. I walked into this building and was amazed at not only the size of the building but also at the number of students who were in the building. Then when I reached the trombone studio I couldn't believe how many trombonists had made the trip to Indiana for the auditions. All these kids literally thousands of high school trombone players would be competing for just a small handful of spots in the incoming freshman class of 2004.

I was standing in the hallway after warming up and just visualizing the performance I began to get excited and become tense. This would be the most pressure I'd ever encounter while performing and it was the performance with the least amount of people listening. I was listening and amazed at how well all these other students played. If you were auditioning to be in the IU School of Music, you were the best player from your high school and you were talented at getting around the horn.

As the time got closer for me to go inside and play for these three outstanding musicians, my heart instantly began pounding. More so than ever before. Here I was, after seven years of playing trombone and trying to become a Master of It I was auditioning to my dream school for a dream position.

I remember how when I walked in the room these three individuals who would be judging me seemed to be your average trombone professor. I think I had kind of put them up on a pedestal thinking that they would be different but to my liking they were just like me. This would help me to calm down and perform as I'd feel less pressure. I'm sure that there were other students standing outside the door and listening to me play, but that didn't bother me at all. I was able to capture the moment and become part of the music. I lost all thinking of what was going on in the real world and became the piece of music. For those of you who play classical music, you probably know what I'm talking about here. It seems as if time just stops and the music takes over. What a great feeling.

I would finish the performance and then proceed to do some sight reading for them. Sight reading is something in which I have always excelled in. I can quickly visualize the notes on the page and then put them into my head, then convert them from my hand to my arm to tell me what position to go to on the trombone to play that note. This was always fascinating to me as I struggled with memory in some other areas of my life, but for some reason when it came to remember or being able to quickly sight-read music I was nearly a genius at it. Sight reading comes in handy in several situations. Not only in auditions like this but when one is a professional musician sight reading is something you may be asked to do on a consistent basis.

Looking back on this phenomenon now, I can conclude that my ability to sight read at nearly a perfect level was probably attributed to my having Asperger's syndrome. You see, Asperger's can affect a person in several negative ways, but it can also leave a positive impact on someone. It can give and often does provide someone with a gift and most often a very inspiring gift. One that can even provide inspiration for others.

Importance of looking past Negative Affects and Finding the Positive.

While it's easy for a person on the spectrum to sit around moping about the negative effects that Asperger's Syndrome or Autism has on them, I believe that it's important that the individual realizes that there are several positive traits to having Asperger's or Autism. There have been a great many individuals with Autism who have gone on to live very inspiring lives. Some acquiring PHD's, some running businesses, some providing counseling services, and some just by being creative and using what they have as a gift. I also believe that it is extremely beneficial that the friends, family, and professionals living and working with the individual on the spectrum recognize these qualities that are positive and unique about the individual and feed that back to them. There can be nothing more helpful to the self-esteem than to have someone tell you something positive about yourself. This will give them a little more self-confidence and hopefully motivate them to work a little harder at developing these great qualities and using them as a gift.

Special Interest and Inspiring qualities can lead to many great things.

In my opinion, there are a great number of things that an individual on the spectrums special interest and positive/unique qualities can lead to for them and others. One of which could be helping them find a job. By using our special interest, we can gain employment. If you can find a career field that has something to do with your special interest, you will be an expert at your job. No one else will be able to perform it better than you. So, this is another reason why it's crucial not to discourage someone from having a special interest even if it seems a little too intense. It will be more intense than a NT's normal interest level. This intensity is what will allow them to become an expert at something in which they are good at and can use to help not only them succeed in the world, but to educate others.

What happened After the Audition?

After leaving Bloomington and heading back to Huntington

I felt good about my chances. I really performed the solo the best I had ever performed it and was thrilled with the way in which it came off to the trombone faculty. The trombone faculty seemed fairly pleased with my playing and asked me some good questions in which I was able to answer maturely and properly. I left feeling good about myself and my performance.

When I got back home to Huntington and went to school the rest of the year would fly by. I would be so extremely busy with show choir competitions, Fort Wayne Youth Symphony, teaching some trombone lessons of my own, working at Ponderosa, and yet still trying to find time to practice. Yes, even if I got into IU, it wouldn't mean that my work was done or that practice time was over. In fact, my work would just be beginning. I would be expected and want to practice even more and at a more intense level. I was excited about the opportunity that I had and was hoping that I would be accepted and get the chance to make the most of it.

Show Choir Competition Season 04

In 2004 the Huntington North Varsity singers would have what I thought to be "the most successful" season out of all four of my years. We seemed to have developed a great sense of style and the band really blended well with the singers to create an amazing sense of blend and balance and a terrific sounding ensemble. It was a very memorable musical experience. We would win every competition but one that year. At the end of the season we would make the trip down to Indianapolis and compete in the North Central competition. This would be the toughest competition that we'd ever competed in in all four years I was in the group. There was a group nicknamed, "Attaché." This group was from Clinton, Miscopy?? They were supposedly the top ranked show choir in the country with the Varsity Singers consistently being in the top five or ten choirs in the country. We were extremely excited about the chance to compete with this group and really wanted to beat them.

Show Choir competitions would make for extremely long days. They consisted of a morning or early afternoon performance in which every choir would have the chance to perform and show what they had. Then there was an afternoon awards program in which they awarded special caption awards such as best instrumental ensemble and best stage crew. They also occasionally had a best performer award. Then after announcing all those caption awards they would pick the top six scoring choirs to go on to the finals in the evening. Each of the six groups would perform again in the evening in an order that was determined by a random drawing.

We would often travel to places far away to compete in competitions. I can recall a few times in which we left at 6:00AM on Saturday morning and didn't return home until 3:00 or 4:00AM on that Sunday morning. These would make for very long and tiring days. At the North Central competition, I had the honor of going up to the stage to accept awards after the end of the morning/afternoon performances. I was excited for this because I would get to go up with two girls. It was a custom that the guy and girls would lock elbows, so I was able to have a girl on each side of me which meant so much to me.

I must admit at this competition I wasn't really expecting us to win best band and I knew that winning grand champions at the competition was going to be a challenge. To my surprise when the gentleman read "and the best instrumental ensemble goes to.........." The Huntington North Varsity Singers, I was stunned. I was so happy as we had just beaten the top show choir backup band in the country. This band was so good that the band itself had a nickname. They called themselves "The Sound Machine."

After winning best band and having a moment to celebrate that it would be time to get back to business. Something that I want to point out quick here is that for me, when I had something that I was passionate about going on that was going extremely well for me I completely forgot about the social world and all the negative experiences that came with it for me. It was like an escape goat. This is the reason in which special interests are so important because they become a way of therapy for the individual on the spectrum who's dealing with rejection and coping with autism. Special interests in my opinion could be the best source of therapy for someone on the spectrum if there are used properly.

At the end of the first round of competition we found ourselves in an unfamiliar spot. We were in second place a few points behind Attaché. We didn't often have to come from behind to win a competition but if we were going to pull off the unbelievable upset we would have to come from behind. To pull this off we would need to have our best show of the season. If not the best show of our lives. We were calm and confident. In fact, as I can recall I think the parents of the students in our group were more nervous than we were. I think they were so nervous and wanted the championship for themselves more so than we (the students) wanted it. This would put the students under a tremendous amount of stress. In fact, I can recall that the entire week leading up to that competition the parents were driving us nuts because they were in there pushing and pushing and talking like we had to win. Trust me, the kids in varsity singers wanted to win, but at that point in the season everyone is drained both physically and emotionally.

The End of an Era "Final Show Choir Performance"

Here we were, late in the evening hours of the last Saturday in March of 2004. We had come to the point in time in which the senior class from Huntington North High School was to perform at their last show choir competition. We were in the finals and playing catch up with Attaché. The seniors I'm sure had mixed emotions, and I was just excited to play. Show choir was amazing to me because of what we call "dance breaks." Dance breaks are just that. The singers stop singing for a brief period and just focus on their dancing. The goal here is for the singers to show off their amazing dancing skills, but the band often thinks the goal is to play as loud as humanly possible in this situation. These dance breaks would be some of my favorite moments in high school and to this day they are still some of my most sacred and favorite moments. The focus was on the singers dancing, but we were so loud it would be quite difficult to ignore the band.

We performed our hearts out that night only to find out that it just wasn't quite enough. Attaché, from Clinton, Mississippi was just too good. While we managed to sneak out of there with the best band award in the morning session, we would fall short group. This was the only competition we lost in 2004. After finishing in fourth place there was a lot of disappointment from the kids but more so from the parents themselves. I think we had kind of spoiled the parents of the group members in previous years and then earlier that year by winning so much that the parents had a harder time dealing with defeat than the students did.

When the awards were over, and we retreated to the room to get ready to leave I'll never forget something that happened. You see everyone who had been involved with the group knew that winning best band was exciting and an accomplishment but winning that and not coming in first place over all meant nothing. While we band members knew that we could be excited about our accomplishment we understood that there were more important tasks to be accomplished at these competitions. Well, one of the newest band members who was just experiencing not winning grand champion at a competition for the first time in their life came back to the room and was yelling and screaming and celebrating because we'd won best band earlier that day. He didn't know why everyone was so down and depressed. Well he got some dirty looks and that was one time to where I didn't feel like I was the only one who was out of place.

NT's can and do make mistakes

I think that often most people think that the NT's in the
world are perfect communicators and have no social
problems, but I don't think this is true. I think everyone
has social problems. Socializing is just something that's so
unpredictable. While those of us on the spectrum make a
lot more social mistakes than our NT counterparts it is
important for us to remember that even NT's can struggle
from time to time. We shouldn't get too down on ourselves
for making mistakes. This is damaging to the self-esteem
and it doesn't do anyone any good.

Springtime has arrived (Spring Musical and more.

The ending of show choir season would bring one of my
favorite times of the year. With the season ending in mid
to late March, this would mean that spring time was right
around the corner. This would also mean that my birthday
was coming up very soon as I have a March 27th birthday.
Birthdays were always such a drag to me. I mean I had
great family and the support that the family would give me
would be incredible, but I was missing something. Most of
the time kids going through school often have birthday
parties not only for their family but also a party for their
friends. Often you would invite friends over to eat some
pizza and just have a good time. I would often try to
accomplish this feat but often no one or at least very few
would show up. I know that my mother tried extremely
hard to put on parties and try and get other children to come
play with me. For some reason to which I had no idea why,
no one would want to come to my party. Again, I

attributed this to the fact that I was fat, ugly, stupid, and worthless. Those thoughts can be so hurtful to one's self.

Other kids at school would often pass out party invitations but they would pass me up as they didn't like me or didn't enjoy hanging out with me. I can recall wanting to be invited to someone's birthday party so bad, but it just wasn't going to happen for me.

Spring Musical

The spring of 2004 would also be the first time that Huntington North would put on a musical in which a pit orchestra was needed. For my first three years they did musicals that didn't require pit accompaniment but this year they were putting on the musical "Seven Brides for Seven Brothers." This would end up being a good show and once again I enjoyed myself playing my trombone. For those of us on the spectrum we really find it relaxing to be able to enjoy our special interest.

I wouldn't have much luck in the socializing world during the musical either. Attempts to develop good friendships would fail and I'd once again feel rejected. Eventually I'd get to the point to where I just put friendships and pain altogether in the same sentence. Trying to make friends equals pain. It would become a bad thing to me and at times I'd often try to stray away from people as often as possible.

The much-awaited decision

It was mid-April on a warm day when I came home from school to find a letter in the mail from the Indiana

University School of Music. I was excited, anxious, and nervous all in one. I was prepared to handle the outcome no matter what the letter said as I had a few other choices in mind for a college, but Indiana University was at the top of my list. As I opened the letter my hands began to shake. After reading the letter saying that I had been accepted as a trombone performance major to Indiana University in Bloomington, Indiana I let out a huge sigh of relief. This was what I had wanted. This is what all those countless hours and hours of practice had led to. This goes back to one of my favorite sayings I got from an old professor of mine. It's a rather obvious statement but it's so true. The statement is, "hard work pays off."

I immediately started to spread the word to everyone in my family that day and I couldn't wait to spread the word to my music teachers at school and everyone who had been a huge inspiration in the music world for me. I felt so blessed to have a chance to pursue my dream of becoming a professional musician. I was ready for the next chapter of my life to begin and excited about the musical opportunities that would be presented to me. I was however still concerned with my social struggle to find friends.

Wrapping up a High School Career with Prom and Graduation.

The end of May had arrived, and it was officially the end of a very challenging journey for me. A journey that was filled with some ups and downs, mostly downs. While I had had some success in the music world, I'd really struggled with academics and especially social relationships. I was still dumbfounded as to why I had such a hard time making friends. It was beyond my comprehension as to why no one wanted to be a part of my life. Why didn't a girl like me? Why didn't guys think I was cool like they were and want to be my friend? I had so many questions that had not been answered socially that I was just hurt and confused. I couldn't wait to get out of Huntington and get to Bloomington as I thought maybe it was just the area I was in. Maybe only the people that lived in Huntington hated me and I would meet some people at Bloomington who would accept me for who I was and like me. I was trying to stay positive and I just thought that maybe someone down there would accept me.

Before getting a chance to leave Huntington in what I was sort of hoping would be for good at the time I'd have a couple of more high school events and a summer of working at Ponderosa to get through. Normally events such as prom and graduation were meant to be meaningful and something that a high school student should enjoy for the rest of their life. Unfortunately for me, due to my unusual circumstances these events would be miserable and stressful. Everything socially was so hard for me to understand and I would spend time over analyzing it and beating myself up over any mistakes I'd made or at least mistakes in what I thought I was making. However, I didn't really realize that these mistakes were directly related to social unawareness due to having Asperger's syndrome, but I knew that something was wrong. There was something a little "off" about me that other kids just didn't like.

Prom

In the weeks leading up to prom I became really stressed out. There wasn't much going on for me to worry about as far as grades, or auditions, but I was extremely worried about finding a date for the high school senior prom. This was extremely important to me. In the previous year's I'd missed out on nearly all the Christmas dances that we had at our school and I really wanted to go to prom with someone. I had decided that if I didn't have a date there was no way I was going to take a chance on showing up there without a date and getting made fun of by my peers. I even had a plan ready in case I didn't get a date.

In fact, I had a plan put together in case I couldn't find a date. I didn't want to just stay at home and not go to prom because I wanted my parents to at least think I was successful in getting a date. I wanted them to think I was successful in at least finding one friend in high school. To them getting a date wasn't hard. They would often wonder why I didn't show any interest in girls in high school and so did many other people. I was often asked on occasion by people if I was gay since I never had dates or even hung around girls.

Being asked if I was gay was the most frustrating thing in the world. No, I wasn't gay but due to my poor social skills it was easy for people to assume that. In fact, I was completely the opposite. I loved girls. There were more than a handful of girls in which I would say I thought were the most beautiful and amazing people I'd ever known in my life while in high school. It wasn't that I didn't want

anything to do with them at all but more so that I didn't
know how to have anything to do with them. At least in the
way in which they wanted. Any attempts to try and talk a
girl into going on a date with me would lead to rejection,
being made fun of, and ridicule which would completely
ruin my self-esteem. In each attempt I'd make to get a
girlfriend my self-esteem would drop a level due to the
girl's reaction to me. Their reaction was like "umm wow?
You like me? You of all people? How could that be?
You're the most fat and ugly guy that I've ever had ask me
out. You're pathetic and should be ashamed of yourself for
asking me out." Now obviously I don't think they ever
quite said it in those words but unfortunately that is what
they were implying to me whenever I tried to develop a
relationship with them.

After spending a couple of weeks trying to salvage a last-
minute attempt at a date, it was Monday of prom week and
I had pretty much thrown in the towel and given up on
going to prom. I had my plans all arranged to drive around
on that Saturday night so that my parents would think that I
went to prom. I just didn't want them knowing what a loser
I was. I was going about my business during the week like
normal, practicing trombone, working at Ponderosa and
doing some end of the year things at school. I had decided
that there was no hope for me in getting a date for prom. In
fact, I'd decided that I was just stupid, and girls hated me as
well as guys. Where did I belong I'd often wonder?

Social unawareness of people on the spectrum

I'm going to use this as an example as to just how socially

unaware or uneducated people on the spectrum are. I for one was one that just didn't comprehend basic social interactions and didn't know how to interpret them. For example, when I was younger whenever I wanted to go on a date with a girl I'd just walk up to her and say the words, "hey, I think you're really beautiful and incredible and I'd like to get to know you. Would you mind going on a date with me?" I don't think I received one single yes when I tried to ask girls out like that. But to me that made perfect sense. If you want to go on a "date" with a girl, then you should ask her to go on a "date." It wasn't until much later that I learned that dating was more of a game than it was about two people having emotions and feelings for each other. Well it's not just a game, there are emotions and feelings involved but it seems like you must play a game of being hard to get and toying with a women's mind to get her attracted to you. This whole dating concept is still very confusing to me and we'll be talking much more about this later.

I would get made fun of by other guys so often due to the way in which I would try and ask a girl to hang out with me. I didn't understand the meaning behind playing hard to get with them. Today it seems like to me you almost must imply that you aren't interested in them, but you are interested in them at the same time. This philosophy makes no logical sense to me and it frustrates me like none other. This leads me to another good point about logics.

People on the spectrum often take things to be very logical. For example, in my situation when I wanted to ask a girl to go on a date, it was logical to me to simply ask her to go on date and that's what I did. Unfortunately, I should have had a more illogical approach. I'm still working on learning how all this works but people on the spectrum will often take anything you say very literally. So, it's important when you know someone who's on the spectrum that you are very careful with things you say and make certain that the individual understands what you're saying. Again, we will devote a whole chapter to this later in the book.

A pleasant surprise

I would often always be the odd man out in a group of people. This was the case at lunch during all my middle school and high school years and it was no different on my senior year. However, on Monday or Tuesday of prom week a girl who I ate lunch with had her boyfriend breakup with her. I remember how sad she was and feeling so bad for her. She had her heart set on going to prom with this guy as they had been together for quite some time. She seemed heartbroken, so I thought I'd offer to take her to prom. At first, she wasn't too thrilled about the idea and I think she was holding out to see if she could find a hotter date but eventually on Wednesday of that week she called me at home and asked me if I would go to prom with her? This was a miracle and I was amazed because I didn't even really have to do the asking. I simply just offered. I had a prom date and I was going to try and make sure that she had the best night of her life. Unfortunately, it would prove to be a very difficult task.

her life. Unfortunately, it would prove to be a very difficult task.

This girl was an extremely beautiful young woman and she even played the flute in band. I was bound and determined to make sure that she had a good time at prom. I quickly began planning as I went to the flower shop and ordered a corsage and a dozen roses for that Saturday. The next couple of days we would spend talking about what we wanted to do for prom. She was still very hurt and upset from earlier in the week when her boyfriend decided that he was going to dump her. To this day I'm not sure why a guy would ever dump a girl with so many great qualities.

I know if it were me and I were ever lucky enough to have a girlfriend like this girl, I would cherish her, respect her, honor her, and do whatever it would take to make her the happiest woman in the world. I feel that a woman deserves to be cared for like she means the world to a guy.

We had decided that we were just going to eat dinner here in town at Applebee's. Nothing too fancy as it was such a last-minute thing. Up until that Wednesday evening I hadn't even planned on going to prom. So, we went to Applebee's, but we did this in our regular clothes. We decided that it may be best to do this instead of wearing our prom attire and taking a chance and spilling something on it.

We then would go back to her place and change for the prom. I remember that working the Friday night before and for a couple of hours on the Saturday morning was a very anxious time for me. I had never really had the chance to hangout one on one with such an amazing girl. I wanted her to have the best time of her life at prom.

After a great dinner we would then go to her place and change clothes. I was getting excited. Once we were ready we took some pictures at her house for her parents and then went off to my house to take some pictures. I was so happy to be doing this as this meant that my mom and dad would see me with a girl. Just maybe, they wouldn't think that I was a loser for never being around girls in the past.

Once we left my place we headed over to Ponderosa Steakhouse where I had worked during high school to take some pictures and to show off my beautiful date to the people that I worked with. I had told them all that I had an amazingly gorgeous date for prom, but they didn't believe me. So, when I showed up with her they were in awe. Later, they would ask me how I pulled that off and I ended up telling them how it just sort of fell into my lap and I got lucky.

This would be a night in which I felt good about myself. Not only was I (in my mind) trying to save the day and rescue a beautiful woman by taking her to prom) but I also for the first time in my life was enjoying myself in a social situation with an extremely beautiful woman who had an outstanding personality.

After leaving Ponderosa we went on to meet up with her best friend and her boyfriend. We would hang out at their place for a while and take some more pictures. We took some group pictures as well as individual couple pictures. After picture time it was finally time to head off to the prom at the school. I was as nervous as I had never even danced before. I remember being afraid that I was going to step on her foot or something. But even with being anxious about all of that I still wanted to have a great time and I was just amazed to have such an awesome date.

As we walked into prom I had noticed how couples were holding hands waiting in line. I remember being confused to if I should do this with her or not. Now that I've learned a few basic social things, I'm glad I didn't try and do this as it probably would have ruined the entire evening before it ever even started.

As we got inside I was amazed to see how our high school just had been transformed into a magical place for a dance. We got inside and picked a table and started to chat a little bit with the other people in our group. We then proceeded to get some refreshments and hit the dance floor.

My First Dance

I had only been to one other dance before this in my entire life and I can't remember dancing with anyone when I was there. So, this would be my first real dance of my life. I was nervous but at the same time I was excited. It wasn't as hard to slow dance as I thought it was going to be. In fact, I quickly learned that if I imitated her I could do well at it.

Just How Amazed Someone on the Spectrum Can Be About the Smallest Things

What I am going to talk about now will most likely seem a little strange to the neurotypical individual but to those of you who are on the autism spectrum of things, you'll know exactly what I mean. To someone who has not had any amount of success socially at on in their life just to be able to accomplish the simplest task can be the most meaningful thing in the world to them.

I had this interest in girls in which I know think is one of my "special interest." But to have this interest in girls and being really attracted to certain ones for most of my life to finally be on a date with an extremely beautiful girl to me was like being on top of the world. Being with her that night made me feel special. I can't really describe the feeling to you other than by saying that it could possibly be like you having your first child or you are getting married. To me it was the most amazing and wonderful thing that had ever happened to me in my life.

While dancing with her I had another special moment occur for me. You see, I'd never touched a girl anywhere in my life. Not even on her hand. Well while dancing gentleman are supposed to put their hands on the woman's waste. While this would more than likely mean nothing at all to someone who has done this time and time again for me to be able to just put a hand on her waste was like a dream come true. I was in awe of how beautiful she was and how amazing it felt just to be in that moment. I think some guys would kind of take these little things for granted in a woman, but for me even the tiniest thing is cherished as you never know if you'll ever get to experience it again.

We spent some time dancing and I was having the time of my life, but something just wasn't right. She didn't seem to be enjoying herself too much and I understood why but I felt bad that she wasn't having a good time. I wanted to try and fix it so that she could enjoy her senior prom. I remember trying to engage her and get her to dance for a while, and she did dance but she just wasn't there in the moment. Of course, I knew why but still I would feel horrible.

I remember one of her great friends trying to convince me that it wasn't my fault at all that she was having a bad time, but it was probably strictly since her long-term boyfriend had broken up with her on Monday or Tuesday of that same week. I still felt bad though as I just wanted everything to be okay for her and for her to have the time of her life at her senior prom.

To this day I still wonder if she had a good time that evening. We would end up going our separate ways before the evening was over due to circumstances that were out of our control. I was so privileged and honored to have had a chance to take such an amazing woman to the senior prom and I enjoyed every moment of it. While I do wish that I could have saved the day a little better than I did and made sure she had the most amazing time she'd ever had in her life, I realize that this would have been nearly impossible due to the events that had occurred earlier on in that week.

Later, in the following week I would get a thank you card from her for stepping in and taking her to prom. This made me feel good about myself as I had done something nice for someone to make a difference in their life. I still have the card and the prom pictures stored away in my room as memories of the greatest day of my life. To this day this is one of only two or three women that I'm in a picture with. (Note: I've been in pictures with a few other women since then but there would be other things that contributed to those pictures such as the woman being drunk.) I will talk a lot more about this in a later chapter.

Final week of School, High School Graduation

Well the time had finally come for us seniors to take a walk across that stage one last time. But before doing that there was one me thing that I would get to do that I really loved about Huntington North. Every spring the choir program at Huntington North hosted a spring concert. It was tradition that at that spring concert the show choir would reunite and give one last final performance of their competition show from that year. This was exciting as there was no pressure as far as competing and we could just perform the show and have fun while doing it.

It was often a goal of the band at these spring shows to do something that would be of surprise for the singers such as playing a tune a little bit faster than it was supposed to go and watching them try to keep up with the dance moves on stage. This was entertaining to me as I would get to see it all. I had always had every show memorized from top to bottom and I wouldn't even need to look at my music. I could have left the music to the show at home and still played it nearly perfect.

Of course, at the time I had no idea why this was. I just considered myself lucky to be someone who had a good memory in this area. Now that I am very much aware of my diagnosis I can attribute this great quality to the fact that music was always a special interest of mine. As we know, when someone on the spectrum has a special interest they tend to become a master in that area. They will be able to tell you things about it that no one else had ever thought of before. This is such a great quality to have. Again, we just must be sure that the special interest is an appropriate one.

The spring show in 2004 was a huge success. We were finally done with show choir. I'd never again get the opportunity to play in a group quite like this. While there are a few colleges in the area that have shown choir's that use back up bands like are used at the high school level, most of college show choirs either do not use back up bands, or they use a condensed sized band. This is okay and show choir can still be entertaining, but I would argue that when you have live music and a backup band the intensity level of the show increases and makes for a much more entertaining show.

High School Graduation

If there was ever such a day that could be a huge transition point in someone's life, it was high school graduation day. This is the case for anyone and not necessarily just people who are on the autism spectrum. High school graduation day is a time to reflect upon the past. While looking forward to the future.

For most kids, reflecting on the past meant not only looking back at their previous academic and athletic achievements as well as their extracurricular activities at school. It was also a chance to sit around and reflect upon the special memories of social relationships. It was a time to look back and reflect upon the friendships that had formed. It was also a time to look back and reflect upon any relationships you'd had with a significant other as well as special bonds that you had formed between teachers in school. It was a time to think back to elementary school and remember your favorite teacher in those early years. Thirteen years, a majority of your life to that point was coming to an end and it was time to celebrate the ending of an era but also celebrate a new beginning and the future that was ahead of them.

For me however, it was mainly a time of reflecting upon the past successes in the music world. Since I didn't have very much success with building social relationships, I was more focused upon the successes in the music world. Out of all the awards I had won in high school for playing solo's at ISSMA contests and all the soloist awards at jazz ensemble competitions, the most memorable award for me was being accepted into the Indiana University School of Music.

Of course, another more memorable event that did happen socially for me was attending the high school prom with Mary. This would really stick out in my mind as an event that would provide meaning to life and it helped motivate me to move on at the social level and try to develop friendships even more. Without this one sort of positive success I think I probably would have given up at that point and quit trying. It provided the inspiration that I needed to stay motivated.

I remember that there were so many people there for graduation and I didn't felt a little overwhelmed. As we marched in I was very aware that it was the end of an era and a new beginning. We would receive corsages to wear during graduation and I had a hard time putting it on. I was also having another problem. It seemed difficult for me to balance and keep my cap on. I'm almost positive this had a lot to do with sensory problems that can be associated with having Asperger's Syndrome or Autism. But at that time, I just felt like a helpless loser.

The Handshaking Conspiracy

Luckily my cousin was able to help me figure out how to handle this problem and fit in somewhat. I was extremely nervous about walking across the stage at graduation. For some reason I wasn't very good and coordinated at shaking someone's hand. I would get nervous and tense as I wasn't sure how you were supposed to know what hand the other person was going to put out and when exactly they were going to put it out. I wasn't sure when they were going to be ready to shake hands, and I wasn't even sure how hard they would want to squeeze my hand or have me squeeze theirs. This is often something I over analyze and don't enjoy doing due to the amount of stress it causes me. It's not that shaking hands at all is a bad thing and in fact shaking hands doesn't bother me at all. It's everything that must happen before you can shake the person's hand.

For NT individuals who aren't on the spectrum this is something that they can do with ease and without even thinking about it. It's like they have been programmed as to exactly how to do it. They don't have to think through the steps that someone who has Asperger's Syndrome or Autism may indeed have to think about before they can extend their hand to shake someone else's. I think there are at least five crucial steps to this process that someone on the spectrum must think about or analyze before they shake.

How do I know what hand the other person wants to use for the handshake?

When exactly do I extend my hand out to shake his or her hand?

How do I know how hard to squeeze the hand of the person I am shaking hands with?

When do I let go of the other person's hand?

Where am I supposed to be looking when shaking the other person's hand?

Not only do I have to think about this thing, but I must think about them in detail and consider all possibilities that could occur. This isn't something that I just think about and do. It's something I must think about, analyze and then do. For NT's this whole process can take them two to three seconds. For me it can take ten to twenty seconds before I have analyzed the situation and am ready to shake someone's hand. This creates a little awkwardness for the NT individual as they aren't quite sure how to react to it or what to do while they're waiting on me to extend my hand.

Socializing Can Be Exhausting

For people who have Autism and Asperger's Syndrome socializing can not only be stressful and confusing, but it can very well be exhausting. It's exhausting because the individual must think about so many things that are going on within a social situation that their brain will just become worn out and exhausted. I don't know if there's been a study done on just how much brain capacity an individual with Autism or Asperger's Syndrome uses in social situations as opposed to how much a neurotypical individual uses or not. I would venture to say that an individual on the spectrum uses at least five to ten times as much as the neurotypical individual. This is a study I would be curious to pursue. I plan on doing some checking into this within the coming months.

As we will talk more in depth about later, for people on the spectrum any social situation can be very demanding and exhausting. There are just so many things for us to think about that the neurotypical doesn't even have to think about for a brief second. It's like someone being an engineer. They are an expert in their career field and don't have to think too difficult about something that has to do with their job. But if you were to bring an accountant in to do the engineers job, the accountant would have to spend a lot more time thinking about what to do and more than likely wouldn't be able to be very successful at accomplishing the tasks.

Socializing works a lot like this. Neurotypicals are come preprogrammed or pre-trained in the socializing profession. They aren't necessarily born with these skills, but they are able to acquire them with very little effort in their childhood. Meanwhile we have people on the spectrum whom for one reason or another were unable to acquire these social skills during childhood. It's kind of like neurotypicals took a class in school on socializing that wasn't offered to the people on the spectrum. Imagine if you were put into a job or profession in which you knew very little about and expected to perform at an outstanding level with little or no problems at all. You would probably be scared to death, as feeding your family and your basic survival would depend upon how well you performed. It's no different here. People who have Autism or Asperger's Syndrome are put into a job or a profession with no training and no knowledge of how to perform the duties and skills necessary to succeed at that job. The profession is socializing and while I do know that this is not an actual "job" so to speak, the profession itself seems very challenging and overwhelming to the individual. It's like the accountant being thrown into the engineer's job without any training and without ever even having a college course in engineering. What's going to happen in this situation? Most likely unless the accountant is a genius and somehow has superior skills that are very rare, they would fail miserably.

Socializing is a job, career, and profession.

While we wouldn't typically think that socializing is a job or career because it's not something that we receive a paycheck for. I mean, there's no pay involved in walking up to someone and initiating a conversation with them. We don't get rewarded with pay if we say "hi" to someone. The neurotypical individuals out there probably don't even perceive socializing to be much work at all.

But let's look at this for a minute. Socializing is a tool that is used in a variety of ways. One of which is to go to an interview for a job. If a person has good enough social skills and great work history, as well as references they will more than likely have a chance at getting the job. After obtaining the job, the individual must then use those basic social skills that he or she has acquired over the years to perform the job. While there are some jobs that don't require socializing to be successful most of jobs have some sort of socializing involved. I mean a product can't be produced or sold if no one is doing any communicating or talking. Therefore, it's necessary to have good social skills to excel on the job.

Not only are these so called social skills necessary for performing the job description, but they are just necessary for surviving in the work environment. Employers who often aren't educated in autism will not realize that an autistic individual may have trouble fitting in or getting along with the rest of society. They will more than likely come across situations at work that they are even unaware as to how to handle. This can cause tremendous discomfort. This could either lead to the person on the spectrum getting fired or even quitting on their own due to the amount of stress that the social situations have presented.

This will cause the person to receive a horrible reference and create a substantial amount of difficulty in acquiring another job. This is where I would argue that socializing is a career. Or at least the ability to be able to excel at socializing is a key to unlocking a successful career and obtaining a good job.

I remember many times throughout my life in which I've felt like other people knew something I didn't know about socializing. It's like they had received training in social skills from an early age that I just didn't get the chance to encounter. Maybe they'd had courses on it in middle or high school. There was just something about my abilities that were different than mine. I was often frustrated about this and I would try hard to figure out exactly what the difference between them and I was.

I so desperately wanted to obtain the skills that they had but had no idea how to. At the time, I didn't even realize that my problems with succeeding in making friends and in talking to girls were even related to social skills at all. It wasn't until after receiving my diagnosis that I was able to put two and two together. I had just assumed that people didn't like me because of the way in which I looked. I remember many times in high school where I would wish that I could look like someone else. I wish I could be someone else at times.

However, the social skills gap between the NT world and the Autistic world causes numerous concerns in survival for the person who's on the spectrum. Unfortunately, we live in a world where money is necessary for survival. We autistic people on the spectrum are eventually forced to come out of our make-believe world and enter the real world where it's necessary to gain employment so that we can earn money to help provide for not only ourselves, but also our family. There are many people on the spectrum who can get married and start a family. However, to do that one must have a full understanding of themselves and be okay with whom they are and their diagnosis.

Therefore, when we are forced into uncomfortable situations in places of employment in which we are unable to fit in or always be appropriate we are unable to keep a job. This puts us out of work and back on the streets. Therefore, I believe that getting the people who are on the autistic spectrum to get the adequate social skills training is extremely beneficial to the person on the spectrum surviving and obtaining a career that is worthwhile.

I also believe it would be beneficial if we could somehow educate employers on Autism and Asperger's Syndrome. This country's constitution says that all people in this country are to be treated equal and given a fair chance at employment opportunities. We are not to be discriminated against based on religion, race, color, or in any other shape or form. This would also include that we aren't to be discriminated against based on having a disability.

You can quickly see the significance of social skills and employment. Without social skills, there is no chance of succeeding in most jobs. Therefore, social skills should be taught at a high school and university level. They are just as important to an individual's survival as studying their major in college. Without the basic social skills, knowing everything in the world about your major could possibly not be enough. You must be able to understand how to communicate what you know.

The Hidden Curriculum.

I have often wondered where other individuals have learned all the social norms and rules which are supposed to be used in our culture. Where did I miss out on this in school? Somewhere at some place, at some time a teacher had to teach me about social skills, somewhere right?

This isn't the case. Unfortunately, social skills are taught in what I call the hidden curriculum. There is not a single class in middle or high school to where these kids are taught how to say something, or when it's appropriate to say something, or how to say it. There's no class that teaches them how to read body language or nonverbal communication. It's all done on instinct.

They can just do it as if there's nothing to it at all. I mean it just flows for them. Yet it's such a struggle for me to know how to say something sometimes or even just to look someone directly in the face or eyes. It takes a tremendous amount of courage and effort on my part to even sustain a conversation. I've gotten to the point to where I know how to say hi to people. However, at times I feel as if I'm hurting someone or disturbing them by saying hi to them.

Summing up the problem.

To sum up the problem of what I call the profession of socializing I would simply conclude that neurological people are more equipped to obtain a career in a field of their choice. Unfortunately, at this time only 20% of people with Asperger's syndrome employed, with 12% of them in part time employment. This means that only 8% of people who have Asperger's Syndrome are successful at obtaining careers or full-time jobs.

I must point out that this has nothing to do with the individual's inability to work. It has nothing to do with that at all. In fact, I would strongly argue that many people with Asperger's Syndrome would be some of the company's best workers. The problem however, is within the profession of socializing that is a crucial tool in obtaining and finding a job. Let's put it this way. You can have a bachelor's degree, a master's degree or even a PHD, but if you are missing that one small piece of the puzzle then you will not have your life completed and you'll be miss just one important piece that could be the key for making it all fit together.

Those of us on the spectrum often refer to life and autism as a puzzle. In general, I'd say that everyone refers to putting together their life as a puzzle. Some people are missing more pieces than others. Eventually everyone finds all the missing pieces and completes the puzzle. Unfortunately for people with autism, that one missing piece will often be the only piece that's not there. I've spent many years trying to find this piece of the puzzle. There were times when I didn't even know or understand that I was looking for a missing puzzle piece but just felt different. But knowing of my diagnosis now, I know that I was different because I was missing that one last final piece in finding success.

The Rest of the Summer Before leaving for IU.

The summer started with my graduation party. I had invited a lot of peers from high school and only about two to three would show up. This was kind of discouraging to me. Usually when kids graduate together in a class of 450 or greater like I did a student would at least have 100 or so kids at his or her party. My party was held at my grandparents' house in Huntington.

Lying associated with Asperger's and Autism

It is often true that when an individual is on the spectrum, he or she will have trouble with lying. This is something that has been common in most Asperger's diagnosis. Not only will the individual have trouble due to believing the lies that the neurotypical individual tells them, but once they believe the lie that the neurotypical tells, they will eventually adopt it into memory and their belief system. Once it's liked inside of someone on the spectrum's brain he or she may not be capable of determining if the lie is true or not.

I'm particularly referring to the lies that a neurotypical individual will tell someone on the spectrum such as, you're not cool unless you drink. "Even worse, you're not cool unless you drink and drive like the rest of us." You're not going to be good enough for me if you don't pay me money to hang out with you."

There are so many fibs/lies that a neurotypical individual will try and tell someone on the spectrum. Because of the social unawareness of the individual on the spectrum they will have an extremely difficult time with this concept. I know for me in my life, I've person bought into the fact that it's necessary for me to pay people hundreds and hundreds of dollars just to hang out with me. I was so socially naïve and desperate that I was willing to do anything to have a social interaction with someone. Even if it was only paying $500.00 to hang out with someone for two minutes, I would have done it and I'd still have a difficult time saying "no" and walking away from the situation. Because I know that if I don't pay them to spend time with me then there's not a chance that they're going to become my friends.

This is a major trap that our people on the spectrum could fall into. It's very important that others who are involved in the child or young adult's life try to look out for situations like this in which the individual may be getting taken advantage of or believing this lies that the world is telling them.

The Relationship Between Creating a Make-Believe World and Lying.

When individuals on the spectrum spend their entire life trying to learn how to fit in and be just like everyone else it's easy for them to try and change the way the approach getting to know people in hopes that the change made will be the solution to all their problems. This was the case for me. I would spend numerous attempts repeatedly at getting to know someone only to fail at it and have this big rejection looming over my head.

For a long time, I would try the same things repeatedly thinking "maybe next time it will be different." I was holding out that least bit of hope for the longest time.

Eventually as time went on that hope became less and less. Eventually any hope that I had at having a friend or even a girlfriend was completely gone and I'd all but given up.

As I have discussed earlier in this book, people who are on the spectrum will often retreat to a safe place in which they feel that no one can hurt them. After being rejected so much they'll end up using their imagination to retreat to this little make-believe world that they've created all in their own head. They will feel much safer and less vulnerable there. As I mentioned earlier, I do believe that there are many advantages to this but also some disadvantages of this happening and some things that we need to be aware of.

Imagine that you were someone who didn't fit in and you wanted to know how to. What would do? I know myself, I've did Google searches to learn how to make friends or even get a girlfriend. Unfortunately, these advertisements that will often come up on internet sites saying, "How to get a girlfriend" are often scams and they really aren't intended to help you, sadly enough they're just in it to take your money.

Sometimes people on the spectrum will spend their entire life wondering why they don't fit in or why no one even wants to talk to them. Eventually one gets desperate and decides to try and do something about it. You begin trying to change some things about yourself. You change what you do, how you do it, when you do it, to what extent you do it, and you change so much more.

I was frustrated to the point to where I would try and read

lines of what to say to people off the internet. I tried to pick up on some conversational skills from a few websites and "change my vocabulary." In doing this, I'd try a new thing or two and quickly evaluate and realize that they didn't work either. So, then I'd go back to the internet and find another technique I could use and try again. I was doing these things over and over while still having no success in social relationships with peers. This became so frustrating and tiring.

Losing Yourself

After spending countless days, weeks, months, and even years of trying to change and mold yourself into something (you're not) that will be accepted by society, eventually the individual can become confused and lose track of who he or she really is. This happens because you've tried to mimic so many people and learn from them that you've changed who you were. You no longer remember who you are, what you originally stood for, and what your purpose is in life because you've spent such a significant amount of time trying to fit in and become someone you're not just, so people will give you the time of day, and if anything, maybe so they won't abuse you verbally, emotionally, or physically. After spending so much time trying to be someone else I forgot who I was and what I stood for.

When this day happened, I started to forget what the truth was. I couldn't remember who I was, what I liked, or why I liked it. Everything that was once a part of my life was no longer with me because I'd decided to let it go or change it into something else so that I could get someone else to like me. Trying to change who I was and become someone in which at that time I thought was better than me was a setback to developing myself and my own self esteem. I needed to be spending my time trying to become more accepting of myself instead of trying to change who I was to please someone else.

One day later in my life when I was terribly depressed and miserable and kept trying new things to try and figure out exactly how to be "cool" or liked by other students my age, I just lost it and started bawling in front of a bunch of people. Someone pulled me aside and made the following comment to me, "You don't know who you are, do you?" Wow, this comment couldn't have been more accurate. I had no idea who I was. I had no clue as to who I was because for a year or two now I'd been trying all these different things and techniques to make friends. I had tried so many different things, approaches, and styles that I'd completely forgotten who Travis was and how Travis would approach a situation. I became a "book." Whenever I had a social situation come up I no longer said, "ok Travis, what should I do in this situation." Instead, I said "okay, now what would this book tell me to do in this situation." I spent so much time trying to recall what the book would tell me to do in this situation that usually by the time I thought of what I was supposed to do the situation was gone and not in front of me anymore.

What I thought would be the end of my first job. Leaving Ponderosa.

Towards the end of August, I would start packing up some

of my things to head to Bloomington. I was still working forty to fifty hours a week, so I didn't really have a whole lot of spare time. I also had to keep practicing trombone and piano so that I could become an even better musician and have an advantage when starting school in September. I remember that whole summer people pointing out to me that I practiced too much and that I didn't have a life. They would tease me and make fun of me. I would try to blow it off, but I'll have to admit, it was starting to really bother me. I was glad to be getting away from Huntington and trying to start a new life socially down in Bloomington. I wanted to keep the music aspect of my life, but I knew I had to get rid of the horrible social life that I had experienced here and try and re-establish a better social life in Bloomington.

It was August 18th and my Ponderosa career would come to an end. I would run hot bar for one last senior night with the girl that I'd usually run it with. We were both headed off to college and this was both of our last night's working there. We had a good time and the night went smoothly and I must admit that it was kind of hard to say good bye to the place and a couple of the adults there. But I had to; it was time to move on with life. I thought, surely there are better things ahead. There must be some friends to be made down in Bloomington and life could only get better from here.

After the end of the summer I would spend my last week in town preparing for transition. I began to make some phone calls and get acquainted with the trombone faculty down at Indiana University. I would set up a lesson with my trombone professor Mr. Peter Ellison. I was amazed when I first met him as he was such a fine musician. He had played for a few years with the Seattle Symphony and well he knows his way around the trombone.

I moved into my first apartment the week before classes started. My cousin would help me move in as he has a huge truck. I couldn't believe the amount of people who were already in Bloomington a week before classes had even started.

I thought getting into Bloomington a week or so early would really benefit me. Not only socially but musically as well. I was looking to start my social life over and I thought I'd spend a week or two doing this before classes started. I also wanted to get accustomed to my new surroundings and the new buildings.

There were so many changes to become accustomed to. I couldn't believe how beautiful the campus was. I had normally been down to visit in the winter time and this was my first late fall to early fall visit. I was impressed to say the least. I wanted to get down there and find out where all my classes were. I also wanted to spend some time preparing the orchestra audition pieces. I knew that this was going to be a challenge.

The time had finally come for me to be a college student. I thought that this was going to be an exciting experience and be completely different than being in high school. I was very much looking forward to the change and figuring out how to make friends. I thought for sure that I'd be able to make some good friends in the music school. I thought that maybe through common interest I would be able to just have some friend's kind of fall into my lap so to speak.

After spending a week down at Bloomington getting things organized in my new apartment and figure out how to get around town and mainly around campus, I was all situated. I thought that I'd come home for the weekend to say a few good byes to some family here. At that time, I thought I was going to be saying good bye to them for quite some time as I had no intentions of coming home until Thanksgiving. Little did I know at the time just how fast my plan would change.

Summing Up Pre-College Life from Two Different Perspectives.

Before I move on and talk about what happens in post high school life and adult hood I wanted to take a moment and kind of provide some insight from two different viewpoints on my life here up until this point. In perspective number one I will tell you what was going through my head at the time of heading down to Bloomington, Indiana to start college as a trombone performance major. This will provide insight on what I thought was going on in my life without even knowing that I had Asperger's Syndrome or anything wrong with me.

With perspective number two I will look back at my life from where I am now and provide insight to what I think was going on with me as far as all the problems I was having. This is going to be a much more educated view point of what I was having a hard time dealing with. As you will find out uncovering the fact that one has

Asperger's or Autism is the turning point. Once one knows he has a problem, he can then go about figuring out how to fix it. Please keep in mind that currently I was nineteen years old and about ready to start my freshman year at Indiana University. I wouldn't receive my Asperger's diagnosis until I was twenty-two years of age. While I knew there was probably something wrong with me or at least that I was having trouble fitting in with others and making friends, I had no idea why or what was causing this. It wasn't until much later that I'd start to get a better understanding.

Creating a Make-Believe World and Escaping into Imagination Leads to Lying

It is often a trait for someone who has Asperger's Syndrome to lie. This would be no different for me at times. I often wondered why I was lying but I just couldn't help myself. Now that I've become more educated about spectrum disorders, I realize that sometimes I was lying without even knowing that I was lying.

Yes, this is a very complex and tricky theory. I believe that someone with Asperger's Syndrome could in fact be lying without knowing they are. This all stems down to the fact that they've spent years trying to make friends and get to know people and haven't been successful.

I tried so hard to be accepted by friends and peer groups that I was willing to do anything. There have been times in my life in which I've tried things that I'd have never even thought about doing just because someone would tell me, "if you do this, then I'll like you." I spent so much time trying to do what others were telling me was "cool" that I didn't realize I wasn't even doing anything that I enjoyed doing anymore. I mean, if someone would have told me a girl will like you if you jump off a bridge, there's a good chance that I would have believed them and followed through with that action.

I believe that it is through the process of trying to change who we are so often that we lose track of who we are ourselves. There are several combinations that could trigger the lying in an individual with Asperger's Syndrome. Think about how much time someone with AS spends in a different mindset each day. They often get rejected so often that they're forced to spend most of their time, day, and life inside of a little make believe, imaginary world in which they've created and feels safe to them.

I would often read books about how to talk to people or meet people and they would give me some advice or something to try so I'd go out and try it. In trying it repeatedly I would tend to adapt that behavior into my routine to a point. Unfortunately, not everything that you find online is going to be the most beneficial thing for you. (It's very important to make sure that you check the source of the situation before trying to adapt or learn a new behavior that is being taught.

Even if the source is somewhat useful, it most likely wasn't written or intended to be used by someone who is on the spectrum. People on the spectrum will be less aware of the fact that not everything someone says is something that should be used in social interactions. Plus, what works for one person doesn't always work for the other person. Everyone is unique and it's important that the person who's trying to learn social skills learns them in a way that they can adapt them into their personality without changing who they are.

I do believe that there are certainly basic principles should be followed in social interactions. It's these principles that the individual must learn and become familiar with first before they are able to develop them and combine them with their own unique and special personality. Once the principles are learned, the individual should become more familiar and can possibly start becoming a little more socially aware in social situations.

I was able to learn and adapt some basic social principles but when I tried to mix them with my personality it became very difficult for me to distinguish between who I was. If I was using something that I'd read straight from a book, then how could I know who I really was? Unfortunately, though when you're left with no choice but to try anything and everything that's in front of you, you'll make decisions out of disparity that you wouldn't normally make.

Seeking Therapy to Provide Answers

I believe that therapy is a wonderful idea for someone who is going through depression or anything at all. However, as I would find out if the therapist just wasn't aware or trained in autism or Asperger's there's no way that they were going to be able to tell me that I had any form of autism.

I remember going in to visit several therapists. When I

walked in and asked them what was wrong with me I was asked several questions. They wanted to know what exactly was bothering me, so I told them that I thought other people hated me and I couldn't make friends. I told them that I was sure girls hated me and I'd never get a girlfriend. I wanted to know why? I was asking the counselor why no one liked me and why it was so hard for me to make friends.

Immediately these counselors would start drawing conclusions. They would ask me things like, "Are your parents split up?" "Are your parents dead." "Are you adapted?" "Were you abused as a kid?" These counselors would ask me so many questions. At first, I immediately knew the answer to all those questions. No, my parents weren't split up; they were still together and have been for 27 years. No, my parents weren't dead, that was an obvious statement. I wasn't adapted, and I was never abused as a child.

I told a few counselors this and they kept saying well there must be something. Something that's bothering you and holding you back. I swore to them that I'd never been abused nor had any of these problems in my life. They kept suggesting that I probably did when I was younger. I went to a handful of counselors and they all kept saying the same things.

Eventually after visiting anywhere from fifteen or twenty different counselors within a couple of months I started to question myself. I began wondering if maybe some of those things hadn't really happened to me. They suggested that I couldn't remember it because I wasn't wanting to, or I was just trying to deny it. They had me stumped I really began to wonder.

Somewhere along the way counselors convinced me that the problems I was having in social interactions with my peers was because of my parents. They kept saying that it had something to do with my parents. After hearing that so many times repeatedly I began to wonder, and I eventually started to believe it.

I became kind of bitter and my home life started to suffer. Now, not only was I struggling in the social world, but I started to question my parents about things. I just wondered why I was different and wondered if the counselors were right and if something severe did happen to me during my childhood. I kept questioning my parents about what happened as a kid and why they didn't seem to have a lot of social interactions with other people their age.

As time would go on there would be a few counselors continue to harp on the fact that my problems had to be related to my home life. It's highly important that when one is seeking therapy that you recognize that not all psychologists are trained about autism or Asperger's syndrome. So therefore, when you don't realize yourself that you have some sort of autism or Asperger's related problem you'll be easily persuaded into believing that your problem is whatever that counselor tells you they are.

Even once a person has already been diagnosed with Asperger's syndrome it may not be a good idea to just walk in and go to any counselor and say, "hey, I have Asperger's syndrome. Please help me. You would think that this would be okay to do as these people have been put through at least four to six years of undergraduate school and graduate school. Most people you're going to seek therapy and counseling from will have at the least a master's degree in clinical counseling.

I strongly recommend that you search hard and find someone who's already obtained a doctorate in clinical counseling. Even then, there are still a few psychologists with doctorates who may not know what Asperger's Syndrome is. Most however, will be familiar to some extent with autism.

I have visited with several clinical counselors who didn't have much background as to what Asperger's syndrome was and couldn't really help me out much. All that they could do was to refer me to someone else who might. If possible, I would recommend asking ahead of time before you make an appointment with a counselor to see what their background is on Asperger's syndrome or autism in general.

After being passed back and forth between several counselors for about a two-week span in my life, I finally started to believe what they were telling me. Somehow, I gathered from everything in which they were saying that I had somehow been adapted and my real parents were dead. Somehow, I created that out of what they were telling me.

I believe that it was possible for me to create this because I thought that these individuals were well respected individuals and would know everything and I should believe and trust them. Between them telling me that they thought that something had happened in my childhood and me having the characteristic and ability to create my own imaginary/make believe world, I started to really believe this scenario. I thought that I had been adapted and my real parents were my adapted ones.

This is not the case as now that I've became more stabilized over the past couple of years I've been able to do some reasoning for myself. At the time though I totally had myself convinced that I was adapted, and my parents had died in a car crash somewhere along the line. I began telling this to other peers thinking that maybe I would make more sense to them.

Eventually I kept thinking more and more about it and becoming more and more miserable toying with the idea of deciding if I was adapted or not. It was like I was being brainwashed by an outside source telling me that I was adapted, and my parents were dead but at the same time fighting with what I knew from the inside about my parents being real and alive and very non-abusive. It was a rough time though as I was questioning it. I questioned my memory of the events of my childhood at one time, thinking that well maybe I was just too young to remember my parents every abusing me in anyway and indeed maybe that had.

I couldn't tell. I just couldn't get a grip on things and I couldn't figure them out myself. I was lost and confused more than ever and would cry as I went to sleep every night. I was wondering who I really was and why I was here, as well as what I was doing here.

11 A DREAM DASHED

After getting all situated in my new apartment down in Bloomington just off the campus of Indiana University and coming home to spend the last weekend in which I thought I'd be in Huntington for an extremely long time. It was time for me to head back down to Bloomington on Sunday, August 22nd, 2004. Classes were slated to begin on Monday, August 23rd, 2004. I remember being extremely excited but very anxious and nervous. Indiana University was a huge place and certainly I had had many outstanding opportunities to develop friendships with not only guys but girls as well.

I couldn't wait to get down there and start playing my trombone with all these amazing other talented musicians. This was my dream. This was my dream being fulfilled and coming true. I couldn't have asked for anything better than this musically. Socially I was still looking for improvements in relationships with peers and I thought that IU was the place in which this was going to happen for me.

I would get into Bloomington at around 7:00 pm on that

Sunday evening. I didn't have much to do that Sunday evening after getting there except for relax and get used to my new place. I had a great apartment thanks to my grandparents and I had imagined staying there all summer long and taking some summer classes.

As I came into town and began to see the beautiful scenery and realize that this situation was real, and I was not dreaming it up, I began to think about the next few years of my life. I imagined myself making many amazing friends and meeting a woman of my dreams. Graduating with a bachelor's in trombone performance, landing a professional gig, getting married, and having children. I had my life all planned out as to what I wanted to happen. I went to bed that evening feeling the best I'd felt about myself in a long time.

For the first time in a long time I was thinking positive and was motivated to get up in the morning and begin my day. I thought that this was going to be perfect and I was going to be okay. I went to bed that evening and had a difficult time falling to sleep since I was so anxious, excited, nervous, and a little scared all at once. I was in a new place, with new surroundings, and new people but I knew that this opportunity had to be better than being in Huntington, Indiana where peers were always mean to me and no one wanted to be my friend.

The First Day of Classes

After spending the night in my brand-new apartment, it was time for me to get up. I had a music theory class at 8:00 AM and I would have about a half hour to forty-five-minute commute just to get there. Due to that fact that I was unable to live on campus I had to drive to the university's football stadium and catch a bus there that would take me to campus and drop me off near my first class.

After waking up at around 6:00AM and taking a shower, I immediately started doing crunches. Crunches were the beginning of a routine for me that would really interrupt with other important things in my life. I started doing these crunches when I was a junior in high school because I had a cousin who was big into working out. He did crunches every night and would lift weights occasionally. He was big on being in shape and I also wanted to be in shape.

I started doing crunches because I thought that I needed to lose weight. I thought that girls probably didn't like me because I was fat and ugly and it was time for me to do something about it. When I started doing the crunches I was only doing about thirty of them a day. By the time I had started my freshman year at Indiana University I was doing 200 a day. This would take me about five to ten minutes which wasn't really a big deal.

For some reason I noticed that I couldn't make myself do the crunches at night. Originally when I'd started out doing these crunches I was doing them at night before going to bed. As time went on I started having to do them in the morning before I could ever even go anywhere. This wasn't so bad though as I was only doing 200 of them and it would only take a few minutes.

The reason that I had to start doing them in the morning

was because I thought that I was fat and ugly. I thought if I worked out in the morning before I left my house, and anyone could see me that I'd look a lot better and be much more attractive to girls. It got to the point in which I just had to do them. I couldn't make myself not do them. It became an obsession of mine. (Often people with Asperger's Syndrome will also have Obsessive Compulsive Disorder (OCD.) In fact, often people who end up being diagnosed with Asperger's Syndrome are originally miss diagnosed with (OCD.)

This wasn't such a horrible thing for me at the time though as again I wasn't doing anything that would take up a whole lot of my time in the morning. Just 200 crunches and then off to class. For some reason it made me feel better about myself to do this. Whatever the reason, I'm not sure. This is another perfect example here about how someone on the spectrum's behavior is a result of something that is beyond their control.

The Bus Ride to Class.

For my first day of school I really wanted to be early so that I could be sure and catch the bus and get to class on time. In fact, as I did in middle and high school, I would want to be one of the first ones to class. I wanted to get in there and be in my seat before the other students got in there because I didn't want to have to be faced with walking up to one of them and asking them if it would be okay if I sat next to them. I thought that they would get mad at me for even asking if I could sit in the same room as they did. While I was trying to be optimistic about developing friendships I was also realistic at the same time, as I knew what I had experienced before, and I had some reservations about trying to meet new people for fear of the same things happening and being rejected and ridiculed again. I didn't want to experience that painful process any more than I already had.

There were so many students waiting around to catch the bus that I felt overwhelmed. I wanted to retreat and go back home to my apartment because I didn't know how to handle being around all these people. The buses come and pick you up at the football stadium. Now normally a freshman wouldn't have to go through this step to get to class because they are required to live on campus their freshman year.

Unfortunately for me, due to my circumstances, I would have to catch the bus and ride it from the football stadium to the university's main location in which all the academic buildings were. This bud ride was scary for me. I remember being scared out of my mind.

Since normally freshman live on campus their first year and would never be riding this bus until the sophomore and probably most of them their junior year I was the young pup who had no idea what to do or what was going on. These other people on the bus were so cool and I wanted to be like them more than I could explain. They just had a sense of calmness about them, meanwhile I was freaking out.

One of the things that I didn't like about having to ride on the bus like that was the fact that I was a music major and played trombone. So, I had to carry a somewhat good-sized instrument on the bus with all those other kids. It was crazy. I got many strange looks and it seemed like people didn't want me on the bus or they just thought I was dumb and stupid. I'm sure they wondered why I was carrying a trombone on the bus. Most students probably had a locker on campus because they lived on campus or close by to campus, but I didn't even have a locker yet nor did I know how to get one. In fact, I never inquired about getting a locker while at Indiana University in Bloomington. I was too scared to ask someone how to get one because I didn't know who to ask or how to ask them. I would just carry my instrument back and forth on the bus every day that I was there.

Another thing that bothered me about the bus was the fact that there were so many students that would ride it but there were not that many seats. There was nowhere for me to sit down on the bus. I was carrying my trombone and a book bag, and I had nowhere to sit. Now I'm sure that many neurotypical individuals would be quite capable and comfortable of this situation and be just fine with standing there and holding onto the railing or something to that nature. But for me since I had horrible balance issues due to my lack of sensory motor skills trying to stay on my feet while on the bus was a nightmare.

I would often bounce back and forth and run into other students who would get really upset at me and curse at me or tell me to get the f'' off the bus you moron. As if I hadn't had enough verbal or mental abuse in high school. Here we were again dealing with many of the same things.

As I stated earlier in my elementary years I had a bus driver who would start driving as soon as I would get on the bus. He would take off before I would be able to get sat down and I would lose my balance and, on some occasions, fall. My mom would tell you that I was afraid of riding his bus and there was a time in which I didn't want to ride a school bus at all. For me, if I'm to be riding in something it's best that I'm sitting down so I don't roll around. There's no guarantee that I'll be able to stand on my feet on something that's in motion unless I'm sitting. In fact, just to give you an example, to this day I can't balance on one foot for more than two or three seconds before having to catch myself with my other foot. Sensory motor skills have always been hard to control for me and now I know it's because of having Asperger's Syndrome. It's important to get support in this area and there are many ways in which you can try and improve your balance issues. If you have a child that's dealing with balance problems or if you're an adult on the spectrum who has balance issues, I suggest finding a good occupational therapist to help you in this situation.

During the entire bus ride, I would be holding on for dear life. I still had to hold onto my trombone and my book bag. This would create a tremendous challenge for me and I'm sure that to other students it was rather amusing as it probably looked like I was riding on an out of control roller coaster but, yet it was just a bus that was only moving twenty to thirty miles per hour at best. I still had issues and it was completely out of my control. I was helpless. This is another one of those classic situations in which a behavior or action is simply out of the individual on the spectrums control. There was really nothing I could do to help myself stand up on the bus. I had to work extremely hard just to avoid knocking other students over. I often felt bad for accidentally contacting a student on the bus. I felt as if I needed to apologize to them for running into them and I often did.

An Incident in High School that Came to mind in this Situation.

It was during this first bus ride of my life from the football stadium to the campus itself that a situation in which I had encountered back in my freshman year of high school came to mind. This situation back in high school would happen to have been the most embarrassing and worst day of my life. I remember hating myself because this happened. Being on this bus full of college students made me think about this situation again and I wanted to be extra careful so that I could try and prevent it from happening.

Unfortunately, this situation that happened in high school would be caused by "time" or should I say a lack of "time." Time has always been one of my worst enemies. It just seems like people are always in such a hurry now a day. People just don't have the patience to slow down and allow someone the time they need to succeed in life.

The date was Thursday, December 14th, of the year 2000. I was a freshman at Huntington North High school and I was sitting in my Biology Class. Now, unfortunately the Biology class was on the complete opposite side of the building from my locker and the band room. Biology was my fourth period class. Fourth period was my last class of the day because of our block four scheduling.

I always brought my trombone home with me to practice every night. No matter what, my trombone was going to be coming home. This would mean trying to bring it on the bus with all these other students who thought that I was a dork or a geek because I played the trombone. They would often pick on me and make fun of me as soon as they'd see me get on the bus with this instrument of mine. At that age, I didn't understand why they were doing this to me and I didn't attribute it to the fact that it was because of the instrument I was playing and not because of me. I thought that they just hated me and wanted any excuse they could to make fun of me or bully me as well as make me miserable.

I know the day was December 14th, 2000 because I have always been one to keep a journal. This evening when I got home from school I would go straight to my room to grab my journal and write in it. This would be one of those occasions in which I would end up spending nearly the entire evening in my room with only coming out to eat. I wrote about my day and what I had experienced.

As the school day was coming to an end and the bell rang I'd have to race all the way across school to my locker, make sure I had all my homework, and grab my trombone out of the band room before I could even begin to think about heading for the buses. This would prove to be detrimental to me on this evening.

It was a cold, snowy, December day and there was ice on the ground. Whenever I wanted to get my trombone after school and catch the bus I would always have to run to make it to the bus on time. If I wasn't there the bus was going to leave me at school and I'd have to go through all the trouble of explaining to someone what happened, so they would call my parents or someone else in my family to come pick me up. I'm not sure if I would have really known or understood how to explain it to them at that point and time.

So, this day was no different than any other day. I was running to the bus except for this day I would have to run through ice. Unfortunately, I managed to fall on the ice banging not only my trombone on the ground but tearing up my knee. It hurt bad and it happened right in front of my bus. As I was always one of the last students to get on the bus (and I hated that fact), everyone on the bus saw me fall. I immediately got up and limped my way onto the school bus only to hear everyone pointing and laughing at me for being such a dork. I'd fallen on the ground and hurt myself and people were making fun of me. I don't understand why kids would do this to someone. Why couldn't they just see if I was okay? Why did they hate me? Again, I was so fat and ugly that I had just given them another reason for making fun of me and teasing me. I was devastated and embarrassed and couldn't wait to get home and get off the bus that evening.

After finally making it through the bus ride from the football stadium to the main part of campus I quickly got off the bus at my first opportunity. I didn't care if I had to walk further to find my class I just wanted to get off there out of fear of being laughed at or made fun of. I think I would have walked an extra twenty miles just to get out of riding the bus. Being on the bus was just miserable for me and I couldn't stand it. I wanted to be free of the pain of being pointed at and laughed at. I felt bad because I wasn't as cool as these other students.

After getting off the bus on the first day of school I was overwhelmed at how many people there were on Indiana University's campus. Indiana University usually has about 60,000 students enrolled in classes during the fall and spring semesters. I was used to going to school with about 2000 kids but being at a place to where there was 60,000 plus people all trying to navigate themselves around the campus was amazingly challenging.

There were so many buildings and I had a difficult time finding my first class. Luckily there were other people heading into the music building in which I was going to, and I was able to find my way into class. Being one of the last ones in there I would be forced to ask someone if I could sit beside them. I remember being so scared that they were going to say no, and I was going to be standing up during the entire class. I prayed that they would say yes, and I could find a seat. After asking two or three kids if I could have a seat next to them a girl finally said I could and I sat down and unloaded my books and my trombone. Most students didn't carry their instruments around with them, but since I was new and didn't know how to get a locker or didn't even know how to go about asking for a locker I would often carry mine around with me. It wasn't always easy navigating around campus with a huge trombone in your hand since there were so many kids on campus. I remember accidentally running into a few kids and having them turn around and push me or something. Again, I felt like such a loser. I was such a small fish in a big sea.

As I got into class I was amazed at how big the classroom was. There were anywhere between 400-500 students all in the same lecture hall. I'd never seen anything like this in my entire life. It was so overwhelming and stressful for me. But I quickly became attracted to just how talented all these music majors were sitting in this room with me. We could hum pitches and scales without receiving a key and we were right on. This would have never happened in high school.

When you get the best of the best together all in one classroom and sing the sound that you get sounds like you're in heaven. To this day I still wish I could be sitting in that theory lecture hall with all those amazing students. In fact, if I would have been there with them to this day I would have been graduated.

After theory class I had some time to relax and I quickly ran over to the McDonalds that is on Indiana's campus. I would get a quick bite to eat and a drink and sit outside as it was so nice that day. There was nowhere to sit so I ended up standing against a wall. As I was looking around and observing some people I was able to notice that most of the students were congregating in groups just like they had done at my middle and high school's. I was a little disappointed when I noticed this because I was kind of expecting and hoping for the situation to be a little bit different for me down at Indiana University.

I quickly went back into my high school mode of thinking that I was the most stupid and worthless person in the world and that all these people wanted to be friends with everyone except for me. Was my life a mistake? What had I done to people to be shunned and treated like I was a thing and not a person.

I quickly went about the rest of my day on campus. I had a couple of more classes and then I was able to retreat for the walk to catch the bus. The bus was a little more crowded this time as it was late afternoon and people that had signed up for and scheduled late classes were now awake and heading to their classes. While others were going home at the same time. Once again, I'd be forced to stand up with my book bag in one hand and trombone in the other while trying to hold on to the pole all at once. This was extremely hard for me to do and it was so packed that we were shoulder to shoulder. The trombone just got in the way. I remember thinking to myself that maybe playing trombone wasn't such a great idea. Why didn't I play something smaller or better yet, not play any instrument?

I can't remember ever being so excited and anxious to get off a bus in my entire life. Once I was off the bus I raced to my car. I wanted to get out of that parking lot as soon as possible. I was hoping that maybe the next day would be a little easier as I would be getting used to the size and magnitude of the campus. As I got home that evening I immediately started playing trombone. Auditions for orchestra and concert bands were that Tuesday and Wednesday. I really wanted to land a spot in IU's top orchestra. To do this, I'd need to have a flawless performance.

I practiced for about two or three hours and then decided that I was ready. I put the horn away and went out to the swimming pool that was at my apartment complex. I thought maybe I could meet some people out there and become friends with them. Who knows, maybe I would get lucky and meet a beautiful woman who would at least maybe smile at me or say hi to me. Either way I would be in heaven because there would be women in bikinis at the pool. I stayed at the pool for an hour or so without one single person coming over and saying hi to me. Of course, due to my social history I wasn't about to just get up and go over and say hi to anyone at all. Especially a gorgeous woman. I would be way too scared to do something like that.

I came back in and began to read some of my music theory homework. This would be something that I'd never seen before in my life. Again, we had some basic music theory in high school but the kind of music theory that you're going to see in high school is going to be nothing at all like the kind you'll get in college. Especially a college that has such a prestigious reputation as Indiana University's School of Music did.

After spending a couple hours or so studying I fixed a late meal and watched some television. I was worn out. I then went off to bed and found myself unable to sleep as I began to replay the day's events in my head. I just couldn't get over the whole bus scene or how big the campus was. It was astonishing to me that so many people could be in one place at one time.

Sleep problems Associated with Social Stress

For someone who has Asperger's Syndrome or Autism sleep problems are a normal thing to have. It's not because you're not tired or the fact that you have a problem with sleeping itself, but it's due to the fact of the experiences in which you've encountered during the day.

Once the day is over and you've had a chance to wind down and do some thinking you begin to replay social situations in your head. You think about something in which you were made fun of or ridiculed for and try to analyze it to figure out what exactly was done wrong. Once you analyze it and come up with some sort of idea of what you have done wrong (which may be correct or incorrect) you begin to think about different situations inside your head and imagine situations in which you could have done it the right way. This is so intense that it can interfere with your ability to just fall off to sleep. If you're an adult and having trouble with this I would recommend talking to your psychologist or family physician.

Unfortunately, kids who have autism or Asperger's syndrome aren't going to be able to understand or know that this could be a reason as to why they aren't sleeping. They could toss and turn all night and never have any clue as to what kept them awake. I would say that if you're a parent of someone on the autism spectrum that it's important you check in with them from time to time. Just ask them how they're sleeping? If they report to you that they are having problems falling asleep then you could guess that it's possibly due to the over analysis of social events that have occurred throughout the day. This is not something that you will be able to just take away or make it go away for them. There are medicines in which could help and talking to a qualified psychologist would be recommended and preferred in my opinion. That night seemed short. Once getting to sleep I slept well but 6:00AM came very early. The sun was shining, and I was ready for another day. I was bound and determined to make this day be better than the first one.

I started my morning off with my traditional glass of chocolate milk. Since my childhood I have had a tradition of always starting off my day with a glass of chocolate milk. I use white milk but mix it with Nestlé's Quick. If you've never tried this, I would highly recommend it. If I was ever unable to start my day with this traditional glass of chocolate milk due to traveling my day would be horrible. It was one of those things that I just had to have to begin my day. Of course, we know that there are many things in life that someone who has autism or Asperger's syndrome do that are just like this. We tend to come up with a routine and we want to stick with it. Changing it can cause distress and really bother us.

After my morning glass of milk, I proceeded to do my crunches. Once again, I'd complete two hundred of them one by one. I still don't understand why I feel better about myself after doing something as simple as crunches. For some reason it can boost your confidence a little bit. I would need much more than a little boost however.

It was about 7:05 and it was time for me to get in the car with my book bag and instrument and head over to the football field. The night before, I had come up with a solution for my problem that I was going to walk to campus instead of riding the bus; however, it turned out that somewhere from within me I would pull out the courage and guts to attempt to get on the bus again.

Once again there were several hundred students gather around waiting for the bus. My hopes of being the first one to get on the bus were immediately shattered when I pulled in and there were that many people there in line. I thought I was early, but I guess there are so many people that go to Indiana University that I'd probably have had to be there by 6AM to be one of the first ones on the bus.

I was tense and nervous as the bus pulled up. I had to wait a couple rounds though as I was far enough back in line that the first two buses couldn't fit me on. This was bad because I had more time to think about the bus ride to the school. I was simply overwhelmed. I remember visualizing the whole bus ride as if it were a music performance. I imagined walking onto the bus without my instrument and acting cool like the other kids. I imagined that I could walk without having to hold on to something while the bus was moving. I imagined that somewhere on that bus ride there would be some other students that wanted to find out about me and would say hello, or at least smile at me. I was feeling calmer as I was kind of in a dreaming state.

When the bus pulled up I was forced to snap out of my

dreaming state. It was such a good dream that I nearly forgot that I had a trombone and almost walked off and left it. Falling into dream land like that felt good as it was also something that I have been used to doing for a very long time.

I thought maybe the bus ride wouldn't be so bad. Unfortunately, when I walked up to get on the bus I kind of tripped and made a fool of myself. Everyone was staring and of course they were laughing. I'd just provided them with some awesome entertainment so now they had something to talk about on the bus ride to campus. I was frustrated as I got on the bus and ended up trying to lock myself into a corner to where I would be able to hold myself up and not move.

My book bag and trombone kind of grazed a couple of people and I got a few dirty looks. I didn't say anything at all as I never did, and I looked straight at the ground. I wanted to get off the bus so badly, but I couldn't for just a few more minutes. During that Tuesday morning bus ride, I decided that I was going to leave my trombone in my car every morning so that I wouldn't have to carry it around all day. I thought this would make the bus ride easier and more comfortable for not only me, but everyone involved as well.

This would of course mean that I'd have to ride the bus an extra time, so I could go back to my car and pick up my trombone and then come back to campus with it. While I hated the bus, I thought the tradeoff would be worth it so that's what I would do from now on.

I got off the bus on Tuesday morning and had to search for some new classes. Most colleges here in the United States go off a Monday, Wednesday, Friday/Tuesday, Thursday class schedule. Meaning that you had the same classes on Monday and Wednesday, as well as Friday, along with having a Tuesday and Thursday class. I liked this as it gave more time to prepare homework in between each class.

Going into my first college ear training class was quite an experience. There were so many people there. Luckily for me I was musically inclined and was able to keep up with the brightest individuals in that class. We would be asked to do things that I'd never done before. One of those things included singing in front of people. As soon as I found that out I was a little nervous about it, but I knew that I was a talented musician and could most likely handle something of this nature.

What I didn't like was the fact that the professor would just randomly call on people. I'm not sure if this is due to my Asperger's Syndrome or not but I have a hunch it is. I just dreaded to be called on for an answer and this was always the case throughout middle and high school. What if I didn't know the answer. What if I didn't know how to say the answer. I was always so worried about all these little things. Little things that the average neurotypical student wouldn't even think twice about.

I was glad that if it was going to happen in any of my classes it would be a music theory or ear training class. I knew what was going on in this classes and I understood everything. It was those darn education classes such as geology that I would struggle with at times.

I managed to survive the first ear training class and it wasn't nearly as bad as I thought it would be. While there were no opportunities within that first initial class period for me to make friends, I was successful with the musical aspect of it. I was glad to be doing something in which I knew what I was doing. Everything seemed so much easier when I knew how to do it.

The Bus Ride in Mid Afternoon

After the end of my morning classes I immediately tried to catch the bus so that I could go back to my car and pick up my trombone. I wanted to get back to the music building as quick as possible so that I could practice before the auditions that evening. The bus ride to and from the football stadium was a little more peaceful this time as most people were eating lunch.

I quickly grabbed my trombone and waited to catch the next available bus. I made it back to campus with no problems and head for the practice rooms. I spent about two or three hours that afternoon preparing for the auditions and I was happy with how well I was playing. There were just so many talented trombonists at Indiana University that just placing in the bottom of one of their ensembles would be a tremendous honor.

Orchestra auditions were done by a process in which we call "blind auditions." This means that when you go into the room to play for the professors or whoever it is that would be judging you that they are turned around and not facing you. This was good for me because I had enough on my mind without having three amazing musicians staring over the top of me.

I would say that there were probably around forty or fifty of us auditioning to play in the top groups. Everyone would get placed in some sort of a group, but only the top ten or so would be placed in the university's most prestigious ensembles. I tried to listen closely to the individuals performing before me so that I could get a good handle on what kind of competition I was going to have. I was just simply amazed by how well everyone played. I felt like I was in trombone heaven.

There really wasn't a lot of socializing going on at an event like this as they were much like myself in the sense that before a big performance they kind of get themselves in the zone. They really focus in at what's going on or getting ready to happen. This is something that's difficult to do but if you can master this technique as a musician you will be able to go very far in the music world.

The Audition

As the person who was scheduled to go before me entered the room for his performance my heart began pounding. Here I was. It was August 24th, 2004 and I was getting ready for the second biggest musical audition I'd ever had in my life. With the first one of course being my original audition to get into the Indiana University School of Music back in February of that year.

As the kid before me finished up I was ready to go. I was in the zone and I entered the room and quickly became aware of my surroundings. I loved the atmosphere and enjoyed performing. I played the audition pieces down to the best of my ability and they couldn't have gone much better at all. After I finished playing, I remembered how relieved I was to be done with the whole audition process in general. I mean I loved to play trombone and usually didn't mind auditioning for groups at all. It was just a lot more fun to be able to play for fun and pleasure. It was just more fun to be able to relax and enjoy myself while performing music.

Looking back on auditions like that that I've had in my past I'm kind of amazed at how easily it was for me to just go in and perform. For someone who gets a lot of social anxiety and has a hard time coping with that, to be able to just walk inside of a room and play a trombone in front of people in which I didn't know at all and sometimes people that I hadn't even ever met before in my life was fascinating. I didn't understand how this could be.

Now I attribute it to the fact that playing trombone and music in general was one of my special interest. I think special interest can be a great tool of therapy. So not only was I able to calm down and avoid social anxiety in these situations, I was also able to get lost in the moment and fully concentrate on my trombone playing. This would allow me to be even better at trombone and excel in the musical world. This would really allow me to focus in intensely upon the music and it was also a way of therapy. I guess in a sense you could say that this was giving me a way to "escape into imagination."

Wednesday August 25th, 2004

The alarm clock rang, and I was awake and ready for my third day of school. Today I'd decided that I was going to leave a little earlier so that I could walk from the football stadium to campus so that I could avoid having to deal with the crowds on the buses. So, I woke up at 5 AM and had my traditional glass of milk and then proceeded to shower and get ready to go. I finished up my crunches, loaded up the car, and was on the road by 6:30.

As I pulled into the parking lot at the stadium I quickly realized that no one was there. I could just leave my car sit and start walking. I didn't realize how long the walk was. I planned on leaving early enough that I could arrive on campus by 7:30 so that I could get situated and be the first one in the classroom that day. However, to my surprise it took about an hour just to walk to the campus from the football stadium. It was a little further of a commute than I expected.

I got to school and got organized and was in my first class of the day about five minutes early. Luckily, I was able to find my own seat and wouldn't be forced to make someone sit by me. If they were going to sit by me, it was going to be their choice or because they were late and the last one there. I pulled out my books and glanced over some things before the professor got there.

Most of that day on campus was stress free however I was starting to look around and be able to notice how all the other kids were mingling in groups. They were sharing laughs with each other and taking pictures. I'm sure some of them were just getting reacquainted with one another after a long summer. Again, I found myself wishing that I could be just like some of these guys. I started to look for guys who I thought were cool and that girls were attracted to. I thought if somehow, I could learn to mimic these guys and their behaviors I would be as cool as they were and be able to make friends while getting a girlfriend.

Not only were there so many people on campus at Indiana University but there was also more beautiful young woman than I'd ever seen throughout my entire life combined. I couldn't believe just how gorgeous these women were. I wanted to talk to some of them so bad and yet I struggled with even initiating a conversation, so I knew that that was going to happen. If only there was some way in which I could get girls to notice me or just give me a little bit of time out of their day. There was a clarinetist on campus by the name of Sam who was extremely gorgeous. I was attracted to her not only because she was pretty but also because of her unique ability to play a musical instrument.

Audition Results

This would also be the day in which we would find out the results of our playing auditions from the day before. I was nervous about this but thought that I had at least done well enough to place into an ensemble. As I walked up to the sheet I closed my eyes and imagined that I was on the list. As I opened to look I saw my name listed to the IU concert band. I was going to be playing in one of the best ensembles in the country. I was thrilled with this and quickly ran out to call my mom and tell her.

Most people wouldn't understand the magnitude of an accomplishment like this, but for someone who didn't have any success in life outside of the music world this would be huge. Since music was like one of my best friends since I couldn't make real friends, it was like accomplishing something with my best friend. I was now going to be able to play some amazing music and become a better musician.

The rest of that day was spent touring the campus. I thought that I may be able to accidentally meet someone by taking a walk around campus and becoming more familiar and comfortable with my new surroundings. I was able to go to the library as well as the student union where students would often congregate, but once again when they were congregating they were usually in groups of friends and didn't have room for someone else like me. I wanted to have my own group to congregate with so bad. I just didn't have any understanding of how to form peer relationships for some reason. I was stumped, and I would continue to try but things wouldn't get much better.

That afternoon I practiced for a few hours and started to work on some soli for lessons. I signed up for a Thursday morning lesson time which meant that I had to prepare for it on Wednesday nights. In all actuality I should have prepared for it over the weekend and I think I would have if I would have stuck around for a while.

That evening after practicing for a few hours I got on the bus and headed back to the football stadium. It was a lot less crowded later in the evening and I was often able to find a place to sit which made me much more comfortable. I arrived back at my car and loaded it up and took off. I remember that when I got home I would see a bunch of people by the pool and I so wanted to try and meet some of them. So, I grabbed a magazine and took a walk down to the pool. I would sit and read for a little bit thinking that maybe someone would walk up to me and ask me what I was reading. No one ever did walk up to me so after an hour or, so I jumped in the pool for a few brief moments and then proceeded back to my apartment to fix dinner and watch some television.

This routine would become quite common for me over the next couple of days as again for me it was easiest to get into a routine of things and follow the schedule. I had a hard time adapting to change. I just didn't deal with it very well as it took me so long to become used to it. It was stressful and at times caused discomfort. That evening I went to bed early as I was tired.

As I woke up the next morning I found myself a little depressed. The excitement of my first week and my musical accomplishments were beginning to ware off and I was starting to come to grips with the reality of not having any friends to hang out with. I think the fact that the weekend was coming up helped to draw my attention to that. What was I going to do for an entire weekend without any friends or family around?

The next day was much like the first three. This time I forced myself to try the bus once again. Since I was leaving my trombone in my car and wouldn't have to drag it along on the bus for the morning commute I thought it would be a little easier. I was able to get a good grip when holding onto the pole with having an extra free hand. I felt a little more sturdy and safe.

That day at school I focused on schoolwork. I didn't really try to roam about the campus to make any new friends or anything that had to do with socializing. I think I was emotionally drained from trying so hard earlier in the week to find people to talk to or people that would talk to me. I just didn't have any more socializing capacity left in my brain for that week. So, I studied for a while.

I ended up losing my wallet in my breakout group for my music theory class. Luckily for me when I realized I had lost it a couple of hours earlier and went back to find it, it was still there. I was able to get it back and I was glad about that as not having it would cause me all sorts of trouble.

First Official Trombone Lesson

It was on that Thursday morning at 10:00AM that I would have my first official trombone lesson. I'd mentioned how I had come down earlier that summer to do a lesson with professor Ellison before classes had begun. However, this would be the first time in which I'd have a lesson with him in which school was in session. We immediately began to work on some solos.

Professor Leeson had a unique warm up system. He has written his own warm up style that he uses daily and he wants all his students to use it to warm up as well. For professional level musicians warming up can be something that takes anywhere from a half hour to an hour. It's not like high school when players just blow a couple notes and are ready to go. It's much more complex. If you're warming up for a huge orchestra gig you'd better expect to spend around an hour warming up.

His lessons were a little more laid back than the lessons I had taken in high school. It was a completely different teaching style than I'd had before. He was calmer but very serious about what we were doing all at the same time. I think he liked to have fun, but he wanted to make sure that we were getting the work done that needed to be accomplished. This was a quality that I greatly admire in a teacher.

After finishing my lesson for that day, I was done as our ensembles didn't start rehearsing until the following Monday. I went to go back and catch the bus back to the football stadium. I had decided that I was going to spend that afternoon roaming about the city of Bloomington. I stopped for some lunch at Steak & Shake and had a milkshake. I loved their milkshakes if they were just that. I didn't like whipped topping, or a cherry being put on my shake. I then went to the mall to do some looking around. I was trying to find some people that maybe I could talk to. Of course, there were people all over the city and campus in which I could talk to, but I didn't know how to. This was driving me nuts and none of them would ever just come up to me and start a conversation. This was killing me on the inside.

Longing for Acceptance

It was at this point and time in my life when I really began searching for happiness and answers in the social arena. No longer was I okay with putting it off like it didn't bother me. No longer was escaping into imagination and creating a make-believe world good enough for me. Cameron Diaz still made for a great imaginary best friend and I still watched all her movies. I would still sit and watch the movie "Head Above Water." Cameron did a great job of acting in this film and it was one of my favorite movies with her in it. I still want to meet Cameron to this day, not because she's a famous actress or anything like that, but because it would be like meeting my best friend.

It was at this point in my life in where I'd begin to do some searching. I was trying to find a group of people who would accept me. The only problem was there being exactly any groups that were out looking to do a random act of kindness and accept some loser into their group. This would be hard work, but I was bound and determined to do it. It was that determination that would cause me to become even more frustrated. Sometimes I think it would have been best to have not wanted any friends and to have just been able to take my life and accept it for the way it was. Why did I need friends so badly?

Well, I think it's a normal thing for a human being to want and long for friendships. I think we were created to want to connect with one another and build meaningful friendships and relationships. It's just that some people are created with a malfunction in the brain and it makes it more difficult for us to build those friendships. I do believe that the ability is in here somewhere and I just haven't figured out how to tap into it yet.

Home for the weekend!

It was that Thursday evening in which I made the surprising decision to come home for the weekend. Yes, I'd only been there one week, and I was coming home for a visit. I thought that this would just be a onetime thing as I wasn't used to being away for too long yet. So, I went to my 8:00 AM class on Friday morning and then came home to my apartment and loaded the car up. I left that morning and came home and would spend the weekend here. I would end up visiting and hanging out at Ponderosa quite a bit. This was strange to them and me as I remember it was only a couple short weeks ago that I couldn't wait to get away from Huntington.

I would spend Friday and Saturday night at home here in Huntington searching for something to do or someone to hang out with. It was my lack of ability to find someone to hang out with while home that led me to spend most of my weekend at Ponderosa. I didn't exactly want to hang out at Ponderosa when I wasn't working but it was again a place in which I knew people and people knew me and were somewhat friendly to me. It was safe and comfortable when I wasn't working too because none of the other guys could beat me up and the girls couldn't try and take advantage of me by getting me to do their work for them.

For some reason being home and sleeping in my own bed felt safe and comfortable all in one. While there was still no one here that I could connect with or really become friends with for some reason have the family around would help me to be more comfortable and relaxed. I didn't really do much that weekend except for hangout and see my cousin. He had decided to stay close to home here and go to school to at a local university.

After spending the weekend here at home, I would take off to head back down to Bloomington late that Sunday evening. I stayed here in town until about 3:00 or 4:00pm and then I started out for the three-and-a-half-hour drive. The drives for me were extremely peaceful. For some reason I'd always enjoyed driving. I think it was because I was able to have a quiet atmosphere if I wanted one. I could turn the radio off and just cruise with the windows down in the summer time. I loved cruising with the windows down. There was nothing more relaxing than doing that on a bright, hot, summer day.

I made my way back into Bloomington at around 7:30PM. That seemed to be a perfect time to come in. Too much earlier and you would catch the early crowd coming in and then if you waited another hour or so later you'd hit the late arriving crowd. I didn't really have any trouble with traffic rolling in at around 7:30. I had a bunch of unloading to do after getting back from that first weekend. I also had some laundry to do and I'd need to look at a little bit of homework. I had a busy couple of hours in front of me.

That evening before bed I would feel very anxious and depressed for some reason. There was just something that wasn't right. Something about being back there was bothering me. I'm not sure what it was but I just felt crummy about the entire situation. Like I was lost.

Once gain going to sleep that night would prove to be very difficult. I was very nervous about school as the social aspect was really starting to get to me. I just couldn't handle so many people all at once. I began thinking that maybe the school was just too big for me. I now know that this wasn't the case at all but at the time due to my unusual circumstances it seemed like an easy answer as to why I was feeling the way I was.

Leaving Indiana University

On Sunday, September 6th, 2004 at around 8:00 I called my parents. They had just left my apartment about ten or fifteen minutes ago and I was still crying. I was scared to death. I begged my mom to let me come home and told her I'd try to go to school somewhere a little closer to home. After spending about ten or twenty minutes begging her, she finally gave in and told me I could come home. I had never felt so relieved in my life. To this day I'm not sure that I fully understand why I was so scared. I can attribute to the fact that I just didn't know how to fit in with anyone. The only thing that was connecting me with people was my music. Unfortunately, at that point and time my interest in music would not be enough to keep me enrolled at one of the best music schools in the world.

The Long Drive Home

After speaking with my mom and talking her into allowing me to come home, I loaded up some small items in my car and took off for home. I was saying goodbye after just two short weeks in Bloomington. I wasn't sure what I was headed home for or what I was going to do with my life once I got home. I just knew that Indiana University was an extremely uncomfortable place for me and I couldn't bear to be there any longer. I did a lot of thinking that evening on my way home. I wasn't sure why I had chosen to leave and come home because I remembered how miserable my social life was when I lived here for the first eighteen years of my life.

I had no idea what was going to become of my life. Now I was in a situation in which I wasn't enrolled in college anywhere and I didn't have a job. I had got myself into a huge mess. Little did I know that this was just the beginning of a journey. A journey that would involve many disappointments and tragic events. This was the start of what I call "Finding Myself."

Falling to sleep that night.

I can remember that evening being extremely difficult to fall asleep. I couldn't stop thinking about the events of the day and how desperate I was to come home. I didn't understand why I had wanted to be home so bad due to how my school career went socially here. It made absolutely no sense to me.

Thinking back on it now the only thing that I can think of that would have made me so desperate to get home was the fact that I didn't like change. Change was something that I just couldn't handle. This is often the case for individuals on the spectrum as we tend to adapt to and live by a routine. When this routine is interrupted it can cause us severe discomfort and stress.

My brief experience down at Indiana University in Bloomington taught me a few things. I learned that I couldn't adapt to change in a very positive way. My feelings of hopelessness were affirmed during my two weeks. I'd experienced other students staring at me, making fun of me, pointing at me, ignoring me, and I didn't feel as if I belonged there either.

Today, I wish that I would have tried to have stuck it out down in Bloomington. If I would have been able to stay in Bloomington and go straight through school I would have graduate last December of 2008.

Instead, I'm still stuck trying to determine a plan of action for getting me back into school and trying to find an academic area in which I can excel in. That academic area in which I would like to try and excel in is music. This experience down at Indiana University was just the beginning of what would be the equivalent of a nightmare you might experience in a horror movie. The events that would happen over the next few years would leave me depressed and in a very dangerous situation. Without the proper support I'm not sure that I'd be sitting here to tell my story today.

I just can't stress enough how important it is to get help when someone has autism or Asperger's. They just simply can't do it alone. This require so much support not only from family members and or support staff, but I also think that having a good friendship with a peer would be a tremendous help to someone on the spectrum. I know this is something to which I've never had the luxury of benefiting from and I really wish I could have.

12 BIG MISTAKES

The next morning after returning home from Indiana University in Bloomington I awoke to a lot of pressure. I didn't have anything lined up back here at home as far as school or work went. I didn't even know where to begin. I had some ideas though and I wanted to quickly put them into action. (I should note that sometimes people with autism or Asperger's syndrome will often have great thoughts and ideas. Sometimes when we get these ideas into our head we want to act on them right away without thought.)

This was always the case for me. No matter how small or big the idea, I had to act on it fast. Before I chose to attend Indiana University in Bloomington I had strongly considered attending another university closer to home here in Northeast Indiana. Indiana Wesleyan University had been at the top of my list as far as a college choice.

There were many appealing characteristics about Indiana Wesleyan as I had sort of grown up in a Christian background and I did believe in God. I had attended church off and on as a child all the way up until my sophomore year in high school when I started attending regularly. I was attending more regularly in my later high school years since I was able to play on the worship team and use my special interest of playing trombone to communicate with God. I loved to play worship songs of all kinds. From slow, soft, and soothing, too hard, fast, and crazy tunes.

Back in March of 2004 I had went over to Marion, Indiana where Indiana Wesleyan University is located to play an audition for the music faculty there. I was awarded a full scholarship which would help cover the cost of attending school at a private university. It wouldn't come close to covering the entire cost, but it did help to eliminate some concerns I had financially about attending the university.

In April of 2004, I decided to go to Indiana University in Bloomington. When I made that decision, I was giving up my scholarship at Indiana Wesleyan. So, not only was I stuck back here at home now with no job and no place to go to school, Now I didn't even have any kind of a scholarship to help cover the cost of attendance at Indiana Wesleyan.

Another reason in which I wanted to go to Indiana Wesleyan so bad was the fact that a gentleman by the name of Mr. Michael Flanagin was the director of instrumental music there. If you'll remember, Mr. Flanagin was my old middle school band director at Riverview Middle School.

Mr. Flanagin was always my favorite teacher. He was the one who would discover my talents in middle school and help develop me into an even better musician than I was. He put a lot of time and effort into developing my skills. The chance to work with him again in college was extremely appealing to me.

That Monday morning, I would send out an email to Mr. Flanagin over at Indiana Wesleyan University. Indiana Wesleyan was located about forty to forty-five minutes away from my parent's home. I sent an email telling him that I wanted to come to Indiana Wesleyan. I explained to him that Indiana University just wasn't the place for me. I asked if we could sit down and talk sometime and he immediately invited me over that afternoon. I was excited to be presented with this new and amazing opportunity.

Now that I had made a contact and possibly found another school to attend for that fall, I had another fish to fry. I had to find some sort of a part time job. Luckily for me, I had worked for about three to four years at the Huntington Ponderosa and I was able to go in there and talk to the managers and get my job back. While I had never actually quit there, they weren't expecting me to come back and work until the following summer.

They told me that I could have my job back and I'd start working part time immediately the following week as soon as the next schedule came out. This was a huge relief for me. I now had a job lined up and would have a source of income. I then had to worry about where I was going to live. I still had an apartment in Bloomington that was costing me almost $750.00 a month and I wasn't going to be using it. Would I get a place of my own back here at home? Would I try and live on campus at Indiana Wesleyan? Or would I just stay at home with my parents and drive back and forth for this year to Indiana Wesleyan for classes and ensembles.

I wasn't sure as to exactly which route I wanted to go, and I knew I'd have to do some thinking about it before making the decision. I think this may have been one of the last times in my life before I knew I had Asperger's that I was able to take the time and think through a situation. Every other time after that when I would have an important decision to make I'd want to rush into and make the decision in which I thought was best right at that moment. I wanted to be in the moment and do whatever my heart felt was right without thinking things through.

Talking with Mr. Flanagin and being introduced to the ensembles.

It was on that Monday that I met with Mr. Flanagin. We discussed what my possible options were for me to come back and go to school there at Indiana Wesleyan. I had a few options as it turned out. I could try and sign up for classes and start school a week late, or I could just do ensembles and wait on the classes until the spring semester of 2005. I really wanted to start classes right away but felt as if I'd be behind and feel awkward in those classes. I didn't want to walk into a situation in which I had no idea what was going on. I didn't want to risk being made fun of or bullied by other students.

After talking with Mr. Flanagin for around a half hour or so it was decided that I would just take ensembles for the fall semester and then sign up for classes in the spring of 05. I felt comfortable with this decision and I was confident in my ability to be a great musician and contribute to Indiana Wesleyan's ensembles immediately. That same day as I met with Mr. Flanagin I was immediately brought in for ensemble rehearsals. I was excited about this. I was immediately thrown into the duty of section leader of the trombones. This was something that would give me a little confidence boost as confidence was lacking for me those days.

Looking back on things now, with knowing what I do. I think that this may have been another thing that attributed to some social anxiety down at Indiana University in Bloomington. When I got there, I was immediately a young puppy again. No longer would I be the best trombone player in my school. In fact, there were probably several trombonists who were playing at the same level or even better than I was. This was something that would cause some depression for me.

I think the one thing that was able to help get me through high school was my interest in music. Also, not just my interest, but how good I was at trombone. I had something that I was good at and could show to other people. This would always help to boost my self-esteem. It was obvious to me and others that I wasn't the most socially aware kid in school. I was never the coolest kid in school either. But I could play the trombone like no other. This was a positive thing about me. Playing trombone was something to which

I excelled in and being first chair was something that I was happy with. It made me beam with pride. I had a smile on my face most often because I was sitting as section leader in band.

When I arrived down in Bloomington to go to school at Indiana University I was no longer the top dog. While I was still an incredibly talented musician, there were so many people in front of me that I would sit near the bottom of the trombone section in the ensembles. This was what depressed me the most. I think that if I would have been sitting as section leader in the Indiana University Wind Ensemble or Concert band it would have been enough to give me the confidence I needed to succeed in school and stick around Bloomington for at least more than a couple of weeks.

Arriving at Indiana Wesleyan and immediately being thrown into the responsibility of playing first part and being the trombone section leader was just the confidence boost that I needed at that time. I started to try and have more of a positive attitude. I immediately began practicing more and more. I would practice trombone about as much as I did during my junior and senior years in high school.

The Spark Was Back

Being put back into the realm of being one of the best musicians at a school bestowed me with a spark that I hadn't had in about a year or so. During my senior year I had kind of started to lose the drive to succeed in life. Once getting accepted into the school of music I was kind of like, "What more can I accomplish musically?"

Immediately after being accepted into the Indiana University School of Music I would turn my attention back to the social scene or in my case the "lack" of social scene.

I immediately started focusing all my attention back onto trying to develop friendships and becoming obsessed with every reason I could think of as to which I was struggling with peer relationships. I would lose all sense of time and organization as far as school and practicing trombone would go. I spent my days trying to figure out what was wrong with me again.

My lack of spark in life would continue all the way into the fall of 2004. In fact, when arriving at Indiana University in the fall, I noticed that while I was excited to be there, there just wasn't that musical excitement that there should have been for me. I mean the excitement in possibly playing in some of the best ensembles in the country if not the world didn't hit me. I thought that I would be going crazy when I got down there. But I was still depressed. I didn't have any friends and I had never had a girlfriend.

Lack of a Social Life Leads to Depression

For those of us who are on the autism spectrum this is all too familiar of a topic. This is a topic that varies for different individuals on the spectrum. You see, some individuals on the spectrum have no or little desire to develop a great social life. They are completely content with being alone and don't want anything to do with anyone and would rather no one bother them.

Then there are those of us who want to develop peer

relationships and make great friendships with people. Both of us groups are alike in the fact that we have no idea how to go about socializing or developing peer friendships. The difference is in the fact that one group wants to be successful in the social arena while the other group doesn't.

I've recently had the pleasure of meeting quite a few younger people on the spectrum. I've seen my fair share of people that want to connect with others so bad, but don't have the tools to do so. Then I've also seen some individuals who don't have any desire to be included in society at all. In fact, some will do everything within their power to avoid society. Both groups need support and we shouldn't forget about either group.

It is my opinion that even in the group of us that doesn't have any desire for social relationships there is still some need for social and peer acceptance. Unfortunately, what has happened is that these individuals have made numerous attempts to connect with society in the past and have been embarrassed, made fun of, bullied, or ridiculed that they've lost the desire for forming peer relationships. They've put up a shell to society so to speak. This isn't at all because they have no need for social interaction but it's because withdrawing from society and becoming a loner is a much safer and pain free solution.

For the group of us that want to fit into society, life can still become quite miserable. After several attempts to build friendships that lead to rejection the individual on the spectrum will lose any self-respect he or she has ever had for themselves. Their confidence and self-esteem will drop like you've never seen before. Unfortunately, self-esteem is one of those things that's easy to lose, but twice if not three times as hard to build back up.

Self Esteem Becoming a Road Block to Social Success

Once an individual on the spectrums self-esteem has been ruined then we must clear yet another hurdle. It is my opinion that before we can continue teaching our people social skills we must cure their self-esteem problem. There's just no way around this. The saying "you can't expect others to like you until you like yourself" sounds so cliché but it's the complete truth.

Throughout the last few years I've read many articles and books on self-esteem. I don't think there's any one book out there that I've read that really unlocks the secret answer to the question, "How do I build my self-esteem?" Unfortunately, I believe that positive self-esteem develops through positive experiences. This is kind of a hard situation to understand. Because as I said I don't think we can teach individuals on the spectrum appropriate social skills until they like themselves for who they are. So, the self-esteem is a roadblock to teaching social skills.

You may need to consider doing some role playing with the individual on the spectrum in which positive social skills can be learned but more importantly positive comments can be made back to the individual on the spectrum both by the clinical counselor or behavioral consultant and the other people who are acting in the role playing. To me there's nothing more rewarding than hearing someone tell me that I did something right in a social situation.

I think this is because I spend so much time and expand so much energy in trying to learn and comprehend social situations that getting positive feedback makes me feel like it was worth my time and that I'm learning. Doing something right and getting positive feedback for doing it properly goes a long way towards building up my self-esteem.

We must overcome our low self-esteem about ourselves before we can expect to make friends. If you're struggling with this as an adult with AS it's important to find the right kind of therapist for you. There are many things you can do that will build your self-esteem without evening having to see a therapist just for this one thing.

One of those ways is to put yourself out in the world and do things you enjoy. Partake in things that you like doing and things that you are good at. For me, there's nothing more boosting to my self-esteem than to pull out a trombone and whip through a couple of passages. In fact, I've found in the past that on an occasion in which I'm feeling brave and wanting to go out and try to fit in on the social arena, that picking up my trombone and playing a few notes does wonders. Not only does it build up my self-esteem a little because I'm doing something that I'm good at, but it also calms my nerves. Therefore, I will feel a little bit less anxious in social situations.

I'm not saying this will work for everyone but try partaking in something to do with your special interest or something that you really enjoy doing before you hit the social arena. This will relax your mind and allow you to think more clearly out in public. I think it's crucial that we are as relaxed as we can be when we meet new people and begin socializing. Being overly anxious can cause us to make more mistakes than we normally would.

Fitting in with other students at Indiana Wesleyan

As I had arrived at my first ensemble rehearsal at Indiana Wesleyan University I remember being greeted with a warm welcome from the students. They seemed friendly and somehow, they had all heard about me. As one student said, "As soon as you called Mr. Flanagin and told him you were wanting to come to school here, he immediately started running through the halls yelling with excitement. This would make me feel good, as it's not too often in my life in which I've felt like someone wanted me to be around. I thought maybe this was a different situation since these kids were supposedly all Christian students. I thought maybe I'd found my "social" home. I was excited to see how this year would un fold.

I immediately started playing the music that was before me and enjoyed it. I was able to sight read almost anything that was put before me. I never seemed to struggle with a passage of music. I sometimes wish that my social life would have been this simple and something that I didn't have to work at so hard.

After a couple evenings of rehearsal, I'd be invited to go over to the college dinning commons and eat some dinner with a few of the other students in the ensemble. They were trying to make me feel welcome and I really enjoyed and appreciated this. (Note: It seemed like when I would be able to just sit there and not try to develop friendships with someone that people were more welcome to me talking to them or getting to know them. But for some reason whenever I took a liking to someone and started trying to talk to them or get to know them, they immediately withdrew their interest and almost started to ignore me.

The only thing that I can attribute this too is when I wasn't trying they didn't feel like I was weird, psycho, or crazy. However, when I was trying they thought all those things and much more. This confirms for me that the problem I was having was in my approach to developing the friendship. When I didn't try developing a friendship then people at least let me hang around on occasion. But it seemed like as soon as I started trying to develop that friendship with them they would put up a red flag and immediately withdraw. I had to be doing something severely wrong.

Re-acquainting Myself with Ponderosa.

After managing to get myself all settled in at school over at Indiana Wesleyan with just partaking in ensembles and no classes I decided that I would just live at home with my parents at least for this first year. I still had that apartment in Bloomington that I was trying to get rid of. I was anxious to start working again at Ponderosa as this would be something that I was very familiar with and I thought I'd get back into the swing of things with little or no trouble.

A week after returning home to Huntington from Bloomington I was back at work. I started out working only a couple of nights a week but since a few people would quit or get fired I'd immediately get back up to my usual forty hours plus per week. This would be great for my pocketbook and now in September 2004 I still had a decent sense on my head about money.

I was able to save most of the money that I was making and build up a nice chunk of change in my bank account. I only needed to spend about $30-40 dollars a week in gas and about $20 or so in food. This was nice as I was able to save up for things that I wanted and buy them. Eventually I was able to get someone else to take over the lease on my apartment in Bloomington, so I'd only have to pay about two or three months extra rent for the time in which I didn't live there.

Eventually I managed to become the full-time day hot buffet person at Ponderosa. This would mean working forty-fifty hours per week with daytime hours on buffet. I was excited about this as again I was doing something that I was extremely good at. I was learning how to cook more and more things and meeting more interesting people.

Work Becomes a Home Away from Home

Eventually I would be working so much that between working and going over to Indiana Wesleyan for ensembles was taking up most of my time. I guess you could say that work became a nice home away from home for me. I think that this was a good thing because I couldn't just sit around and mope about not having any real friends or not being as cool as the other guys were.

Instead of coming home to mope, I'd get off work and just sit and hangout at Ponderosa. I would order some food in which I got for half the price and try and hangout with other employee's. I never actually developed any friendships that really went outside of the work place, but I think it was nice for me to have people, even if they were older adults that I worked with to just try and talk to or connect with.

Trying to develop friendships at Indiana Wesleyan

It was mid fall of 2004 and I was becoming more familiar with Indiana Wesleyan University. This campus wasn't nearly as big as Indiana University in Bloomington and I felt a lot safer here. I was able to go and come whenever I wanted because it was so close to home. So, whenever the socializing became too stressful I was able to escape and get away.

I would continue to drive back and forth just for ensemble rehearsals. I was in wind ensemble and jazz ensemble. Both groups would turn out to be some of the more fun groups I've had a chance to be a part of. The jazz ensemble played well, and I just love jazz. As I talked about earlier, my parents always used to take me up to Fort Wayne to see the Glenn Miller Orchestra whenever they were coming to town. I fell in love with this group and wanted to play more like them.

The wind ensemble at Indiana Wesleyan University had some interesting opportunities in it. As part of the wind ensemble there was what was called the "Honors Brass Quintet." I was very fortunate enough to be able to play in one of the greatest quintets ever that year. We had great trumpet players, outstanding French horn playing, and a great tuba player. The overall balance of the ensemble was outstanding. For those of you that don't know, a brass quintet consists of two trumpets, a French horn, a trombone, and a tuba.

Another interesting thing that the Indiana Wesleyan wind ensemble had the opportunity of doing was traveling to different churches throughout the Midwest. We had the chance to travel around and use our talents to teach about Jesus Christ to the rest of the world. This was wonderful and as part of this students would be given the chance to do testimonies.

The group usually toured two weekends per semester with an additional weeklong tour in the spring semester over spring break. I would really enjoy traveling and playing and I'd often escape into imagination or find myself in the make-believe world as I was traveling.

I had always thought that it would be awesome to be like the Glenn Miller Orchestra or some group like that and be a part of a traveling band. While, I wasn't making any money to travel with the Indiana Wesleyan University wind ensemble, I found myself often imagining that I was with a group traveling the country performing.

I would also imagine that I was the conductor of the band at times. For some reason, I never had to focus very much on my playing and was often able to drift off into the imaginative state while I was playing. I would imagine being the conductor of a prestigious orchestra. To this day

I love conducting music, in fact you could find me driving down the road and conducting an orchestra at the same time on occasion. This probably isn't the safest thing in the world to do, but it's something I do. I love classical music and I love to conduct.

As the semester went on I was able to use all these musical experiences that I had to help ease the pain of not having a good social life. I began to stop thinking about it so much and was able to focus more on life itself and doing what I wanted to or needed to do to try and become successful in life.

Problems at Work

It was during that late fall of 2004 when I would start to have more problems at work and this time it was coming from the new management. Since we hard poor management and Ponderosa in Huntington, Indiana was losing money, they were often forced to send employee's home early in the day time and leave just one or two employees' around to handle the entire store. I would often be one of those employees who was left behind to run the entire store. It was quite often that the manager on duty would send everyone home but me.

While I understood this, and I enjoyed it as it was quite easy to handle when we weren't too busy but there were those occasions to where we would get extremely busy. Then I would be trying to do cash register, cook the steaks on the grill, tend to the food buffet, and help with delivering the customers food, and trying to keep up on dishes all at the same time.

I remember becoming very overwhelmed at times when we would get busy and feeling frustrated. I think sometimes people on the spectrum get frustrated when we become overwhelmed because we don't have the capability of organizing thoughts in our head. I had a million things that needed to be done all at once and all those thoughts were racing through my brain. But I was unable to organize them, so I often had trouble knowing what I should do first, second, third, and so on.

Unfortunately, this would be a situation in which I was being put into every day at work. I think it's because they knew that I was a good worker and wouldn't complain about it. Again, I think often people knew that I could be taken advantage of because I would take it and put up with it as I thought that it was just a way of life and that for me to be alive and living in the world I had to let people walk all over me and do whatever they wanted to me. This was a philosophy in which I would continue to live by for the following few years as well.

The Empty Feeling

While I now had my life put together in such a way that I had a lot more activities going on and was less likely to be able to over analyze social things I was still feeling some emotional pain. At the end of the day no matter how much I tried to do or became involved with there was still this empty feeling. It's hard to describe it, but it's just like you're not getting any meaning out of your life because you can't connect with the rest of the world. This feeling was one of the most frustrating feelings that I've ever encountered. It drove me nuts.

I had several pieces of my life going but there was this missing piece to the puzzle. This would be what those of us on the spectrum so often refer to as the "missing link." It doesn't matter what you have going for you in your life, if one doesn't have access to the missing link and is unable to complete the puzzle they will probably suffer a great deal of emotional pain and distress.

I had come up with the courage to attempt to make friends at Indiana Wesleyan. This is something that took a lot of courage and a lot of effort on my part. It seemed like I had to work harder at it than other individuals did. I would begin studying things on social friendships and self-confidence. I was reading as many books as I could that had to do with self-confidence and power of positive thinking but unfortunately since this was pre-diagnosis for me, I wasn't reading any books that had to do with Asperger's Syndrome or Autism.

Another key reason as to why the missing link is so important is this fact. I mean, I could read all the books on self-esteem, power of positive thinking, and whatever else was out there but without knowing and understanding that I was just missing a piece of the puzzle or the "missing link" it wouldn't matter how much research and reading I was doing. I wasn't starting at ground zero. I was starting on different floors surrounding ground zero, but I wasn't at the route of the problem.

Without fully knowing and understanding what the root of my problem was it was almost as if I was going through life without knowing who I was. Unfortunately, as I've already discussed, Asperger's Syndrome is such an invisible disability that it's extremely difficult to see the root of the problem.

Girls at the college level becoming young women.

It would also be at about this time when I was only nineteen or twenty that I really became even more interested in women. They say that some people are just late bloomers and I was a late bloomer. I noticed girls everywhere I went. It was like I couldn't avoid them. It was like they were an advertisement that was following me around everywhere.

Indiana Wesleyan University had a male/female ratio of 3 males for every female. So, with me knowing that I was extremely excited as I thought surely with that kind of ratio it would be quite simple for me to get a girlfriend and since these girls were all Christian girls they would most likely be nice to me and treat me well. I was excited.

I tended to like girls who were a part of groups I was in such as wind ensemble and jazz ensemble. I remember as soon as I got to campus meeting a girl named Bethany who was quite a bit older than me. She was a senior and I would be a freshman. She was extremely beautiful though and a very talented saxophone player. She was very kind and easy to talk to, but she had a boyfriend and I think was even engaged so she would be off limits for me.

I tended to get excited when I liked a girl and wanted to focus 100 % of my attention on her immediately from the day in which I would meet her. Then after Bethany there were a few other girls within that Indiana Wesleyan University Wind Ensemble that semester that I kind of formed a liking to. Once again these wouldn't ever turn into anything more than an acquaintance.

I was still a little timid and scared of trying to develop a friendship with a girl since I was teased and ridiculed for it in my high school career. Anytime I would see a girl I liked I would hear voices in my head telling me things that other kids told me in high school. They would be saying, "Travis, you're much to fat or ugly for her." "She's way out of your league." "You would kill her just by looking at her." "She hates you." I heard all kinds of things and these weren't just things that I was making up. I'd had people tell me these things in high school and I believed them. I just thought that there was something wrong with me and I didn't have the right to like someone. So, I had to pretend like I didn't like girls at all, even though I did.

This was extremely hard for me to do. I was one that when I liked a girl wanted to act on it right away and talk to her or ask her out. I would get all anxious and nervous and not know how to control all my emotions. While I was able to control them without making too much of a fool out of myself on occasion there would be times to where I would have to go up to a girl and randomly tell her she was beautiful. I couldn't help it; I just had to express how I felt. I'm not sure why telling someone they are beautiful can be a bad thing but trust me, to some of them girls it was the end of the world for them because a guy so ugly as me was telling them that they were pretty. I think they felt insulted that a guy like me even bothered talking to them.

It was also at about that time in the late fall of 2004 or early spring of 2005 in which I would really become attracted to a girl that I was working with at Ponderosa Steakhouse. This girl too had a boyfriend, but I was confused because every time I saw this girl she would complain about her boyfriend or complain about how he was treating her. I remember that this didn't make sense to me at all. I couldn't understand why you would be in a relationship with someone who wasn't treating you like you were a princess.

At that time, I had no idea how relationships really worked, I just knew that when I saw a girl that was pretty I would get this tingly feeling inside and want to talk to her. Of course, I didn't have the slightest idea as to how to go about talking to her but there was the need and desire there and I just couldn't do it. After struggling with this for a few years now I became frustrated and I just wanted to know how to get a girl's attention.

This is something that I would think about time and time again and it almost became an obsession. I was bound and determined to figure out how to get a girl to at least notice me or say hi to me. I wanted girls to like me so bad.

Unfortunately, this is yet another area where failed attempt after attempt can lead to rejection and ridicule which will immediately lead to ruining one's self esteem. This was the case for me. Attempt after attempt to develop a friendship or relationship with a girl would end in misery and the girl hating me or saying that I was dumb, fat, ugly, stupid, worthless, psycho, or creepy. Unfortunately, while I was and am a little socially unaware and naïve at times I am very much aware of what all those words mean that they were using to call me names with.

But I wasn't trying to hurt anyone, and I couldn't ever understand why girls would feel this way. I never purposely said something or did something to the girl to hurt her in fact I tried so hard to be extra nice to her. I'd do anything she wanted. Basically, I would make myself available to her beckon call.

After several failed attempts I was bound and determined to come up with a plan of showing a girl that I liked her. Since I was unable to communicate with her without her thinking that I was creepy or weird I wasn't sure exactly how I was going to go about doing this. Well one day it all came to me and I had an idea. Unfortunately, this idea would cost me a lot of money and it has never really worked in the way that I had hoped it would to this day.

My idea was that I would send the girl flowers. I would send the girl flowers and write her a note on the card because then maybe it would be much easier for me to communicate what I mean in a non-creepy way to her. So, from that day on whenever I liked a girl, before I even talked to her I would try and figure out how to send her flowers. I would send girl's flowers at school, at work, and pretty much wherever a girl was at that I thought was beautiful. I knew that I would get made fun of or ridiculed for liking her or trying to talk to her but if I could show her that I was a cool guy who was nice then maybe she would want to talk to me.

For me to do this I thought that I would send flowers and a card explaining who I was and that I thought she was a perfect angel and that I really liked her. I would send a dozen roses to every girl in which I thought was beautiful to try and show them that I liked them.

Unfortunately, their reaction to this sometimes was also one of "oh my gosh" what is he doing? Or why are you doing this? But I didn't think anything of it. I just thought that it was yet another failed attempt in trying to show a girl that I liked her and that I would have to try again. So, I would send the next girl that I formed liking to flowers and the same thing happened. I began to think surely one girl will like getting these flowers and want to talk to me and give me a chance. So, I kept sending flowers.

The girl in which I worked with at Ponderosa was a very interesting girl. I liked her a lot and since she was unhappy with her boyfriend I couldn't understand why she was still with him. All she did was complain about him. Well, I thought that I would try and cheer her up by being her friend first. Since I'm not great at talking to people I thought I would do this by sending her flowers.

She really enjoyed this for a while as I think it was something different for her. She would say thank you which made me feel good on the inside. However, she still didn't really want to talk outside of work or develop a friendship or relationship with me. I was frustrated, and I just wanted her or a girl to give me a chance.

It became a routine for me to send her flowers at least once a week at work if not more. Then because I was able to come up with the thought that maybe she would think it was weird that I was sending just her flowers, I started sending flowers to more girls that worked there. I would just send them to them randomly and attach a card saying have a great day or something like that.

Beware: Social Unawareness leads to being misled by peers.

What I am going to talk about next is something that I find very troubling. It's something that happens to people on the spectrum all too often. It's something that we need to educate our people about and prepare them for as they will encounter this at some point in their teenage or early adult years. This is something that I cannot believe is happening here in the United States of America.

What I am talking about is being miss lead about social situations by peers with bad intentions. As I was reading "The Complete Guide to Asperger's Syndrome" by Tony Attwood three months or so ago I came across a section of the book in where he addressed this same issue. As I was reading I couldn't believe what I was reading. The exact same things have happened to me in my life repeatedly. Dr. Attwood has really hit a lot of things in his writing about Asperger's and this is one of the most important ones I believe.

It's unfortunate that it's a fact that we must beware of predators in society who are going to recognize the situation of people on the spectrum and use it against them in so many ways. Not only is it enough for the person to take advantage of us on the spectrum but they also feel such a need to miss lead us and cause us to do things that are even more socially inappropriate.

For someone on the spectrum who already has a hard time fitting in, doesn't understand how to develop friendships, and absolutely knows nothing about talking to girls, it's easy to go to other guys that you see being successful in friendships and dating interactions with women. Unfortunately, this is something I've done quite often, and I can honestly say right now that I wish I would have never sought help from a guy in this matter. At least from a guy in my peer group.

Going back to this situation with the girl from Ponderosa. Well I would often ask other guys working there what I should say to her or how I should talk to her. I would ask them how to get her attention and things like that. Well as I started sending them flowers I was still taking advice from these other guys there that were working with me. I'll never forget that guy who told me some of the most bizarre things, but because I was so naïve I tried them. I tried them because this was the same guy that I would look over and see having three or four girls around him always. He had to know something because he was doing much better than I was.

I remember one day in the winter of 2005 I was talking to this guy about a couple of girls and wondering how to get their attention. I had already come up with the conclusion that since Valentine's Day was coming up in a week or, so

I thought I would send them each a dozen roses or something simple like that. This guy was very much aware of my situation and knew very well that I didn't understand girls or how to talk to them.

He pulled me aside one day and told me that if I really wanted to get a woman's attention that I would have to do something huge and something that would blow their mind. I thought yeah, he must be right "simply because he always had girls around him." He told me that if I wanted to get girls to like me there, that I should send each girl who worked on Valentine's Day ten dozen roses. At first, I was like, wow, that seems like a lot of roses, but he proceeded to explain to me that girls liked flowers and the more they got the happier they were. He told me to send them to every girl who worked on Valentine day, married or not married, as they would simply just see it as a nice gesture and you would get in good with the single girls and he told me I would get some dates.

Getting a date was something that I had very much wanted. I just loved the company of girls so much more than guys. I thought that this guy must be right. I had to do something huge to get a girl's attention. So, I went to the flower shop and ordered as many roses as I could. I think I bought out nearly every flower shop around. I took all their roses. There were eighteen girls working that note so I knew that eighteen girl's times ten dozen roses equaled 180 dozen roses. Luckily at that time I had had at least a little bit of money saved up in my savings account from working so much so I went to the flower shop ready to purchase all these roses.

When I first went to the flower shop I only took around $2,200 dollars. I knew that in the past the roses I had bought for girls ran around $12.00 per dozen. I knew that twelve times one-hundred and eighty equaled $2160.00. As I was checking out at my first flower shop with the first set of roses something happened that put me into a state of shock. The roses were ringing up at a higher price than they normally did. I was wondering what was going on? Unfortunately, I'd never bought roses for Valentine's Day before. I guess that the price of a rose increases rather significantly on Valentine's Day. So now I had found out that each dozen was going to cost me $24.95.

Still very much wanting a girlfriend and believing that this guy who gave me this information knew what he was talking about because he had always had girls around him I knew that this was something that I had to do no matter what the price was. I had to get a girl to notice me in some way. So, I now had to recalculate my figures. After purchasing all the roses my total was $4491.00 or so. This was a huge chunk of money and then after adding in the chocolate I bought for every girl I was up to a little over five grands. Suddenly my savings account had vanished, and I was now down to a little under $20.00 in there.

Flower Delivery Day/Valentine's Day   Monday,
February 14th, 2005

Well after draining my savings account on flowers and chocolates I was excited about the upcoming day. I woke up on Monday, February 14th, 2005 with high hopes of having a wonderful day. Flowers were going to be getting delivered to work and girls were going to have smiles put on their faces. Surely the guy who was helping me out knew what he was talking about. I really looked up to the guy because he was such a cool person with not only girls, but he was also someone that all guys wanted to be friends with.

I worked a double on that day which meant I worked 9am-8pm. I would work hot buffet with one of the girls in which I liked. I had ordered around two or three dozen roses per girl from each flower shop so that meant that at various times throughout the early to late afternoon flower shops would be walking in with between thirty-six and fifty-four dozen roses. I couldn't believe how many roses were there when they came in.

After each of the individual flower shops had their deliver of roses completed there was a restaurant full of flowers. I must say that it was quite festive scenery and an expensive one too now that I'm thinking back on it. But, I was excited about how these girls were going to react because Aaron the guy in which was trying to help me told me that girls loved flowers and the more you get them the more they will like me.

As the girls started coming into work that evening they would be sent into the banquet room to find all their dozens of roses with their names on them. I was able to watch as a couple of them went in there and the look on their face was not what I was expecting at all. They looked terrified and like this was the worst day of their life. I remember thinking to myself wait a minute, you're supposed to like flowers, you're supposed to be happy and love them because Aaron said you would. Why aren't you smiling or running up to give me a huge hug?" It almost looked as if a few of the girls were crying.

My feelings of excitement and happiness had immediately been replaced with feelings of sadness and horror as I could tell that these girls hated me for getting them flowers and chocolate. I had done something horribly wrong again. I was so frustrated and thought that I was such a loser. Meanwhile the rest of the guys in the kitchen were having a good time pointing at me and laughing at me. They would even make comments to me, teasing me. They told me that I didn't get them enough roses and that next time I needed to try at least twenty dozen. (I would end up trying this later and again it would fail miserably.) I didn't get it. My wonderfully amazing day that I was hoping to be the best day of my life had just been turned into my worst nightmare. I was convinced that I was fat and ugly and that girls hated me. Why was I even born, I remember thinking?

A few of the girls did manage to come over and say thank you but even the ones that said thank you did it with such a weird look on their faces that I knew they hated me or thought I was stupid. Later that evening a few guys that were boyfriends or husbands of all the girls that worked there had called in and complained to the manager and said he was going to come find me and kick my Ars. I had numerous guys trying to get a hold of me and I wasn't sure why because I didn't like their girlfriend or wife I was just sending them flowers because Aaron told me that I had to get the girl I liked to pay attention to me.

So now not only had a made a fool out of myself and made girls hate me even more than they already did, but I had also managed to gain some male enemies now. I wanted to give up. I went to Aaron and asked him what I did wrong and again he told me that I just didn't get enough flowers and chocolate. He said next time to try the twenty dozen roses for each girl thing.

Again, for some reason, I was still gullible and desperate enough to try this. Aaron had all the girls in the world talking to him, so I thought that he must be right. The thought that he would be trying to tell me false information on purpose didn't occur to me. The thought never registered in my mind.

I remember going home that night feeling completely worthless and miserable. I was dumb, fat, ugly, stupid, creepy, and a psycho. I was all these things while all I wanted to be was "normal" and fit in with the rest of the people in the world.

The next day was Tuesday, February 15th, 2005, and I had to work a double that day as it was our senior night. I worked 9:00AM to 8:00 PM. I walked in that morning to humiliation and embarrassment as there were lots of people who would just stare at me and ignore me. It was like they were saying "What are you doing?" Or "Why did you do that?" I was so mad at myself and I already hated myself. "Why did they have to go and rub it in" I thought. The manager had called me in to tell me that I couldn't get flowers for any of the girls anymore as he was already fielding phone calls from upset boyfriends and even husbands. The current manager at the time could be kind of a jerk but at the same time also a nice guy. He was like an oxymoron.

Taking Away a Source of Survival

By telling me that I couldn't get girls flowers anymore it really hurt me. You wouldn't normally expect a guy to tell you something like "not being able to give girls flowers anymore is very painful for me" but it was extremely harmful to me. Not having the ability to send a girl flowers with a card was detrimental to my self-esteem and would lead to more depression.

For me, sending a girl flowers and a card would become a way of communicating with her. It was a way of communicating how I felt about her. Since I didn't have the proper social skills to be the biggest flirt in the world and really get her attention like other guys could, I had come up with an alternative to replace that. I thought that by giving girls flowers or a card that I would be able to connect with them more and they would want to talk to me. At least, maybe they would at least know who I was no and say hi to me on occasion.

Now I was even more helpless. I didn't have any source of communication with girls I thought were pretty and liked. I didn't have any way at all to connect with them or tell them how I felt about them. I was rejected, depressed, and miserable. How was I going to talk to girls now? I already don't know how to talk to them in person and now I'm not able to send them flowers or chocolate or give them a card. How am I going to show them I like them?

This would be kind of like taking away someone's special interest. To me communicating with girls had become a special interest and a source of survival. I was reading an article somewhere recently about dealing with dating issues. It said that guys need for sexual encounters with women is not what drives them crazy, but they need to be able to communicate with women on a consistent basis. They really need that social mechanism there to help release those hormones. This article was interesting to me and I couldn't agree more with it.

Eventually after trying so hard to not want to connect with a woman so bad, I was able to quit worrying about the Ponderosa scene so much and became more fascinated by the scenery over at Indiana Wesleyan in Marion, Indiana. I had an "ah ha" moment. I was like "wait just a moment here." There are around two or three thousand girls that go to school at Indiana Wesleyan. All I must do is try to meet them and start talking with them.

I could have girls to talk to, interact with, and send flowers to. I wasn't going to die because I couldn't send flowers to girls anymore. I just had to do it at another place. There were already a few girls that I was interested in over on campus that I'd never even talked to and I immediately sent a couple of them flowers and a card. They were a little freaked out as they had no idea who I was even really. Again, I couldn't understand how they could have been freaked out. I was upset with myself and still wondered why girls hated me. I wanted to get to the bottom of this so desperately. How was I going to get there though? We will come back to this in a later chapter and I'll being to explain to you what my approach was for trying to get there and how I was going to do it.

13 BUYING LOVE

After leaving my job in a sheer attempt to show that I was like everyone else, and was cool, had some guts, and could stand up to people. I returned to school. This time I would be taking real academic classes instead of just the music ensembles. This would provide a little bit of spark in my life once I got past all the anxiety that starting school led to.

I was taking about sixteen credit hours this semester. While most them were still music courses I also had to take some challenging general education courses. I couldn't concentrate very well in my general education classes due to the amount of social anxiety that I was having. It seemed like every attempted approach to make a friend was a disaster and would lead to bad things.

IWU Wind Ensemble

Once again music would be the thing that kept me motivated and trying to succeed in school. I would once again be named section leader of the trombone section which was something that I could be proud of. As section leader I was also eligible to receive grant money for each semester in the amount of $500.00. I couldn't tell if other students in the group liked me too much or not, but after reflecting on this a year or two later in talking with Mr. Flanagin it was decided that they all liked me, but they just weren't sure what to make of me at first. They thought I was a little strange.

While being at Indiana Wesleyan was nice in a way because supposedly most of the students that attended there were good solid Christians. This would make some aspects of life easier but also some other aspects of life a little more challenging.

I was once again a part of the Indiana Wesleyan University Honors Brass Quintet. This was again one of the finest quintets in which I had ever had a chance to play in. There were two outstanding guys in the group; not only outstanding musicians but they were just all around good people. Phil Wiseman is one of the coolest guys I'd ever met in my life and he talked to me and made me feel a little bit included. Paul French was another outstanding musician and another guy who would take me under his wing for a while and kind of lead me along. While to this day, I'm not as close of friends with Phil or Paul as I would like to be, I know exactly what they are doing. Phil is a worship pastor in South Dakota and Paul is a worship pastor here in Indiana.

A lot of time I feel like I'm on a different channel than other people when it comes to trying to build friendships.

My approach is totally different than theirs in intensity. I have a very difficult time knowing when to contact someone you're trying to get to know. Because I don't know when to or how to I'll often drive myself crazy with trying to figure out when the exact perfect time is to text them or call them. This is not good because my anxiety will kick in and make the situation magnify to about twenty times as much as it was. I have a hard time controlling anxiety and it's overwhelming at times.

As I went through the semester I would experience some interesting things. I often wondered about certain social situations and how to develop them and study them. I became fascinated with studying friends. I guess I needed to know exactly how to interact with someone, so I was willing to put a lot of time and effort into figuring it out which would cause my grades to slip and classes to become increasingly more difficult.

I became a little more depressed, but it was this fall that I would be introduced to a high school band director that would quickly become someone I looked up to. I was highly recommended to work on this gentleman's summer marching staff teaching the low brass/trombone section how to play the music for their fall 2005 marching show. I was already busy with school and homework, but I decided that taking on something like this would be good for me because it would look good on resumes and it would help to keep me busy and hopefully less depressed.

I worked their band camp at the end of the summer in August just prior to school starting and this was something that I really enjoyed. They asked me to stay on staff during the fall marching competition season to continue working with the low brass. I graciously accepted their invitation.

I ended up spending quite a bit of time over in Monroe, Indiana that fall. I would drive back and forth two nights a week for rehearsals. It was about an hour drive from Indiana Wesleyan University. I always looked forward to every day and opportunity that I had to travel here to work with those kids. When I was helping kids learn something that I was very passionate about it made me feel important and like someone appreciated my talents and wanted me around. Even if I was 20 and they were high school kids, it still meant something to me to be wanted and included.

I remember that my drives back and forth to Monroe on those evenings were sort of therapy sessions in themselves. I would often put on some of my favorite music and just relax and enjoy the drive with the windows down. I loved listening to marching shows and jazz music in the car. There is nothing more therapeutically for me than listening to music,

Some of the best times of my life were spent on the football field. Both in high school and then again when I was doing support staff for high school marching bands. There is nothing like standing on a football field on a Friday night during halftime of a football game performing a show or even standing on the sidelines watching the younger kids play their hearts out.

Marching band is something that is huge here in Indiana. The kids in our schools have a passion for music and winning. Most groups are extremely successful here in northeast, Indiana. I would travel to Monroe on Tuesday, Thursday, Friday, and Saturday nights which would help keep me busy and not thinking about negative/depressing thoughts over that fall.

School wasn't too bad yet. I was taking basic intro level or freshman level courses. Due to starting college over basically it was kind of like I was still a freshman that had to take beginning level classes before I could get into the real stuff. I remember that I was exceptionally talented at music theory and ear training one. I was always one of the students who knew what the interval was or what the rhythm was. I just hated to be the one student that the teacher would choose to call on though. In fact, there were often when I would want to avoid eye contact completely with the teacher. Whenever I was called on I said, "why me?"

The fall of 2005 would also include going on a couple of weekend tours as an ensemble. I had tried to ensure that I had the same roommates but due to circumstances in which I couldn't control, the other guys who had roomed with me the previous year wanted to room with someone else. This was another circumstance in which I felt neglected because I must not have been good enough or cool enough for them. I wanted to room with them and when I had gotten around to asking them if I could they both said that they were already rooming with someone else. So that left me to basically do a roommate search.

Eventually I would get to know a drummer in the jazz band

who also played percussion in wind ensemble. He was looking for a roommate and we decided that we would give each other a try. He was a cool guy and probably one of the nicest guys that you could ever imagine. It seemed as if he saw something in me that most others didn't and was willing to at least be nice to me.

Sometimes people's actions aren't intentional.

After living through years and years of experiences in which I have been rejected repeatedly by guys and girls, I have concluded that while some people are just mean, arrogant, and rude and will blow you off and purposely ignore you and make fun of you. There are others who may really want to be your friend and connect with you but just as you don't know how to connect with them, they don't know how to connect with you.

This is because both of you have totally different mind sets about socializing. Again, the neurotypical individual has multiple channels of communication within his brain that he or she can switch to at any time almost on instant. Meanwhile the person on the autism spectrum often only has the one basic channel. Therefore, even if the NT wanted to really be friends with the person on the spectrum they would have to work hard at finding the channel in which the individual was stuck on and really bring out that channel in their interactions together.

I often refer to this as if I am a defective television set. Most television sets come programmed with the capability for you to flip the switch and go through several different channels before finding the one in which you want, while the defective television may not allow you to change the channel. Neurotypicals come with multiple channels and are normal television sets. Individuals on the autism spectrum come with one channel and one channel only; we can be defective television sets.

If the individual with Asperger's is extremely shy it will be very hard for the NT to connect with them in anyway. The individual with Asperger's is more than likely going to have many impairments that will delay or affect the way in which he or she processes a social interaction.

Time Delay

Time delay is a major disturbance to individuals with Asperger's or Autism. Time delay is the amount of time that it takes for one to have the initial thought then act on it. For example, I put my hand on a hot burning stuff. My sensory or cans system is telling me that it's hot and burning my hand and without hesitating the brain tells the hand to retreat.

When an autistic individual puts his or her hand on a burning stove it can take a few more seconds before the brain is able to process the thought of, "this is hot, move my hand" which can cause one's hand to become burnt.

As the fall 2005 semester went along I became a little more comfortable in my classes. I still dreaded being someone who the teacher decided to just randomly call on as I wasn't comfortable speaking in front of an entire group at the time. What if I had the wrong answer and they would make fun of me?

Often it would feel like the teacher or professor would pick on me to answer questions though. I think this must have been since I was always trying to look away from the professors and avoid making any kind of eye contact with them at all.

Being a commuter.

Since I still was not able to live on campus due to a bed wetting issue as well as the cost to live on campus, I would be forced to commute back and forth from Huntington to Marion daily. At first this wasn't such a big deal at all as it was only about a forty-five-minute drive to and from school. The only time that I ever wished that I lived on campus during that semester was when I had a 7:30AM class on Monday mornings. It would have been nice to just roll out of bed and put some clothes on and go to class like a lot of kids did.

Dangers of the Internet

It was in about October of 2005 when I was trying to find people to connect with and be friends with online that I would meet a girl. I had joined a dating website in hopes that I would be able to meet a girl and feel more comfortable talking to her online before meeting her in person. I had finally a girl, or at least what I thought was a girl and had gotten to know her and we decided to meet.

She was from Cincinnati, Ohio so I decided that one Saturday afternoon I was going to make the drive down to Cincinnati and meet her. I remember feeling so excited about meeting her. She had emailed me and had instant messaging conversations with me. We texted and talked on the phone once.

When I got there and was supposedly arriving to meet this beautiful woman, there was no woman in sight. It turns out that this person posing as a woman was a man. A man who was desperate for interaction with other men. I was so stunned and disappointed that I didn't even have a clue as to what to say.

I thought "I've got to get out of here this is so weird, and I feel uncomfortable." I have a hard time telling people how I really feel sometimes though because I'm afraid of hurting someone's feelings. I will try and refrain from telling someone the truth if I think it's something that could offend them.

But, I certainly didn't drive the nearly four hours from my home to Cincinnati, Ohio just to meet a guy. I was thinking I was meeting a beautiful woman. I was tricked and fooled into doing something I didn't want to do. This just goes to show you all the things that are out there and how you can get yourself into trouble quickly. I've heard and seen of things happening to neurotypicals but imagine when it's someone on the autism spectrum who could be a little social naïve.

Social Networking Sites

It is my opinion that social networking sites are both very useful for someone who is on the autism spectrum but also very dangerous for us on the spectrum. Imagine being someone who already struggles in social situations. Then suddenly you have this tool called the "internet" that is placed in front of you were all you must do is type and you'll be able to talk to people.

This would both make your life more simple and complicated at the same time. It could make your life simpler because an individual on the spectrum is able to sit at home in front of a computer with no other social disturbances are around and communicate with others. As Dr. Attwood states in "The Complete Guide to Asperger's Syndrome, "when an individual on the spectrum is alone or by himself there is no social impairment. There must be at least one other person there with the individual on the spectrum to cause a social impairment.

The downside to social networking websites is that they can make an individual on the spectrum's life extremely more difficult and challenging. There are so many avenues to social networking sites. There are also so many websites out there for example, Facebook, myspace, and twitter, just to name a few.

Using such websites can be complicated for a neurotypical individual. Imagine how much more tremendously confusing that they can become to someone who has Asperger's. While I do use social networking sites I've had to teach myself the proper way of using them so that I can avoid from coming across as weird, creepy, or psycho.

The problem with sites such as Facebook is that it seems as if they are just adding new applications every day. Facebook for example, started out as a place in which you could connect with old friends by writing on their walls or sending them private messages. When Facebook was first launched it was for college students only.

Today, there are millions of people on Facebook and it is now open to anyone. No longer is it just college students. Plus, we now have the capability to chat via instant messaging conversations directly from Facebook. We have gone from practically zero applications to have literally hundreds of them. Oh yes and they've added the whole status update thing so now everyone in the entire world can know exactly where someone is at and what they are doing. This could be extremely dangerous, and we must be careful about who is seeing our is information.

There was just a story in my local newspaper about how the city is thinking about blocking Facebook from their network. It has been found out that city employees are spending most of their time throughout the day on Facebook rather than doing projects for work. This is another common problem that we have is that social networking sites can become addicting and take away from the rest of one's life. This is not only for individuals on the spectrum but also for neurotypicals. I've known of many NT's who say they just can't get away from Facebook or they don't think they could ever survive without Facebook.

Social Networking 's correlation with "escaping into imagination and the make-believe world."

I have put a lot of thought into this next topic and I do believe that there could be a strong relationship between using social networking sites like Facebook or myspace and "escaping into imagination or creating the make-believe world for people on the autism spectrum. I can remember several instances in my lifetime over the past few years in which this could be true, and it makes perfectly good sense as to how this could happen.

Imagine that you were in your early twenties and sites such as Facebook and myspace are being launched. You have also been diagnosed with Asperger's Syndrome. You've finally figured out that the thought you've had for many years of "something is horribly wrong with me" is completely true.

So, you're suspicions that you don't fit in socially or that peers hate you is finally confirmed. Once again you feel rejected and like you just want a break. You're depressed because you can't make friends and can't get a girl to even notice you. So, what do you do? You explore the world of social networking sites.

Social networking sites allow you to meet people online before meeting in person. They also allow you to do this from the safety of your own home. Unfortunately, when someone has autism or Asperger's syndrome and has been turned down by people nearly his entire life, the fact that you could possibly talk to someone on a networking site is exciting. Once you start making connections via Facebook or myspace and talking to people it can become quite addicting. These people are only here for you to talk to when you're on Facebook. Well what happens when both of you can' be on Facebook at the same time? Then there is no friendship. I have many Facebook friends in which I've never met in my life and I consider them to be sort of like my imaginary friends.

Being in the social networking world may be good for those of us on the spectrum for some time as it allows for us possibly to experience a little bit of social success. With not having to be in person with someone there is no social impairment and we are able to be more relaxed with less anxiety. This could decrease the number of social mistakes that we make.

For someone with Asperger's it may become a way to feel better about yourself. When one is seeing and experiencing positive social interactions via the Facebook or social networking world it would become rather easy for them to just become addicted to socializing via internet. I believe it is extremely crucial to limit the amount of time that one spends socializing on social networking sites. It all goes back to the problem of spending too much time in the make-believe world will cause us to withdraw from the real world and pretty much seclude ourselves into this creative little imaginary world that we've made up.

So, to summarize my feelings on social networking sites, I would say that I think they are extremely useful and helpful for someone who is on the spectrum. I am one who does use them every day. I do however, try to limit the amount of time that I spend on them daily as I'm afraid that spending too much time on them will cause me to become addicted to the make-believe world and its surroundings and seclude myself from the whole world.

So social networking sites are useful for those of us on the spectrum, but they need to be used in moderation and mixed with going out into the real world to try and make real friends with real people. Social networking sites can be a nice getaway and provide one with a huge confidence boost, but again, it's important that we don't over use these networking sites and lose track of our real life, in the real world.

We are Walking and Living Targets.

This is one of the saddest things that I must talk about. Unfortunately, we live in a society in which a lot of people look out for themselves and don't really care much about other people. There are so many individuals out there that will do whatever it takes to get whatever they want without even realizing what it is they are doing to someone. Sometimes I wonder if some people don't ever experience pain.

For example, when a guy tells me that I can be his friend and hangout with him and his group of guys if I pay him a certain amount of money each time I hang out with him, I wonder if this guy even realizes that he may be hurting someone by doing this? To me, it's just a very sensitive area as I really care about a lot of people and I would never ask anyone to give me money for me to hang out with them. If I had ten million people all wanting to hang out with me, I would do whatever it took to make the time to hang out with them without charging them one cent.

I often wonder if these people that have treated me this way in the past have ever even experienced pain in their life? At first when this was happening to me, I thought that they didn't experience pain, but now that I've had some time to think and analyze things, I would say that maybe it's a possibility that they do experience pain. Maybe even more so than I.

I am still trying to come to grips on forgiving some people for some things that they have done to me in my life. I realize that maybe they didn't do them on purpose and they just saw how easy it was and is to take advantage of someone like me. So, they just did it without stopping to think about how it would make me feel. I am working on forgiving them and moving on with my life, unfortunately it's hard for me to get over this and trust some people, especially guys, because there's been a lot of physical abuse from other guys. I think it's a little harder to forgiven someone when the abuse is physical and hurts you.

I think it's extremely important that when working with an individual with Asperger's that we remember to teach them about this and prepare them for situations like this that could come up.

I look back at a few situations throughout my life now in which I could have avoided being taken advantage of if I just would have had the proper awareness as to what was going on. I am the type of person (as so many individuals on the spectrum are) who just assumes that the world is a good and safe place where everyone is nice and wants to help one another.

Unfortunately, as I've learned over the last few years of my life, this just simply is not the case. It's sad but I now must try and remind myself to be on guard and looking out for situations in which people may be trying to take advantage of me or use me just to get something they want such as money, or a new television. I must constantly be thinking about this now when I'm in social situations.

Social situations are already difficult enough for me as I must think and analyze so many different things all at once and it is often exhausting. Now because I've learned that there might be someone out there in the world who's trying to take advantage of me or use me to get something they want, I must also be thinking about being aware of that while I'm trying to make myself present in a social situation. There's just so much to think about at once.

The end of the Fall 05 Semester, Madrigal Dinners.

As the end of the fall semester of 2005 was ending I was proud of myself for accomplishing something in which I had not done yet before in my life. This is something that I should have done a year earlier but due to other problems that got in the way, this would be my first time completing a semester of college and getting college credits. I was excited to have some sort of a record on my academic transcript now. Because my classes were mostly introduction courses that semester I did well in them, so I really set my grade point average (GPA) high. My GPA was a 3.7 or something close to that after my first semester of real classes with real grades.

During the fall semester I had accomplished a lot of great things and some not so great things. I had managed to stay in my classes without withdrawing which as you will soon find out is something that I would later struggle with again.

I also was able to use my special interest and play in as many musical ensembles both inside of school and outside of school. I was in wind ensemble, jazz band, orchestra, and pretty much anything that was musical and included a trombone part, I was in it.

However, there was still this big social situation that was just looming over my head. I still hadn't managed to learn how to develop these peer relationships and I was becoming more and more desperate to find out by the day. I was getting to a point in life in which I realized that any meaning I had in life, with my music and trombone, just wasn't enough. I soon began to discover that the only thing that can provide true meaning in life is having great friendships and being accepted by people around you. Just having someone to say hi to goes a long way towards providing meaning in my life.

The other really bad thing that hurt my feelings during that semester was this guy I had met online from another school. He had said that he was going to be my friend if I did his homework for the entire semester. I did every single homework assignment that he asked me to do and come the end of the semester he doesn't even take the time to say thanks. I never met this guy or hung out with him.

I guess you could say that in a way I've sort of completed more college credits than are officially on my record. I've been told by guys and girls more than a handful of times that if I do their homework for them they will in return be my friend and spend time with me. Each time I have done it and have never been able to say no because I just need someone to talk to me or be my friend. It's just that nearly each time what those other people have told me about how they would spend time with me after I completed their homework for them, they have never held true to their word.

I keep believing that just one day someone is going to hold true to their word. Although I hope that I don't ever fall into the trap of having to pay someone to hang out with me ever again. I can't even begin to tell you how much better off I would be today if I wouldn't have had such a great desire to make friends. If I didn't have to pay someone to hang out with me or be my friend, there are so many things that I could have purchased for myself in which I haven't.

Instead, I've now been forced to file for bankruptcy and rebuild my life. The interesting thing to me is that if I would have purchased "things" instead of trying so hard to get people to hang out with me, there's a lot better of a chance that those things would still be with me here today. The people in which have told me "give me money, and I'll hang out with you and be your friend" unfortunately are long gone. Although, I can't say that it's a complete loss because I wasn't going to be able to afford to pay someone to be my friend for my entire life.

To this day I'm searching and longing for friends that will want to be my friend without me having to pay them money. I'm really looking for people who will accept me for who I am and at least give me a chance to get to know them. I don't understand why I must pay someone to be my friend when other people don't seem to have to pay them money?

Towards the end of the fall semester at Indiana Wesleyan the music department hosts an event in which they call the madrigal dinners. This is a formal event in which people from the community purchase a ticket and are then treated to a formal dinner and show by the Indiana Wesleyan University Chorale.

As part of the show, the IWU Honors Brass Quintet opens for the chorale by playing a few charts. These charts are originals written for madrigal dinners. Some of them were cool and fun to play, while others were a bit more boring. I can remember doing this show well. It was one of the most interesting times in my life.

It was during this show that I would experience what I now know was probably a classic Asperger moment. Unfortunately, because of my love for music, I'd always manage to overbook myself with gigs somehow. The madrigal dinner show was slated for a Friday and Saturday night in mid-December as we would do two shows. On the Saturday evening, I was also supposed to play for a Christmas concert in Columbia City for the Blue River Big Band that I was also a part of. These two places were almost an hour a part. The Madrigal dinners started at 7 and I was supposed to be done and out of there by 8.

Unfortunately, the show would run a little late on Saturday night and I'd be forced to rush to Columbia City. I would make it to my second concert on time, but it was what would happen before that concert earlier in the evening at my first concert that would prove to be an embarrassing moment for me.

As part of the Madrigal theme the brass quintet was all wearing tights. We had all received white tights in which we'd have to wear for both performances. Now this was embarrassing when everyone's wearing the same white tights. Five guys in white tights. However, somehow or another after the first evenings show, I managed to lay my tights down somewhere.

Come about 6:30 on that Saturday evening as I was going to get dressed for the concert I'd realized that I couldn't find my tights. I thought maybe, just maybe I was going to get out of wearing tights that night. They managed to find me something even better than the white tights. Somewhere the costume people came up with a pair of black tights for me to wear. This was entertaining to the audience I'm sure and the other guys would give me a heck of a hard time about this. Looking back on it now. I find it to be humorous and I can laugh about it.

Looking back now and thinking about this situation as someone who now knows I have Asperger's this night made perfect sense to me. I've learned that people on the spectrum will often be very unorganized. Well, I did manage to find the white tights a couple of days later buried under a big pile of stuff in my trunk. I guess I had just thrown them in my trunk after taking them off on that Friday evening.

I would make it to my second concert on time, but it was what would happen before that concert earlier in the evening at my first concert that would prove to be an embarrassing moment for me.

After the madrigals and the Christmas concert with the big band it was time for me to go into my last full week of the college semester. This was going to be finals week and I wanted to ace all my finals, so I could have an awesome GPA and just relax and enjoy my winter break. I remember that studying for tests and finals would be something that was difficult for me. I've always had a hard time sitting still long enough to study for a test. I think it's due to the overwhelming amount of social anxiety that I encounter.

Luckily for me in my first semester these tests would be simple. I managed to get A's on all of them except for one in which I received a grade of a B. I had just finished up my first semester in college without dropping out due to anxiety or depression. I was happy and couldn't wait to head back in January. If I could just focus on things like school and work in life and not worry so much about making friends, then I think that I'd be able to succeed with school and work. It's because I'm constantly thinking about and overanalyzing my social life that I become distracted and can't focus on school or work. But when you're getting taken advantage of and constantly being teased because you aren't like the other students or employees, both work and school would become two of my greatest challenges.

During the spring semester of 2006 I would continue my academic journey. I was excited to have passed some classes and be moving onto a few higher-level classes. I continued my studies in music and tried to play in as many ensembles as possible. Once again, I didn't do a whole lot outside of school. I began really trying to get to know good quality people through the internet. This is something that I wouldn't recommend someone with Autism or Asperger's syndrome do unless they are aware of what they are getting into.

I for one was very unaware of what I was getting into. I would think that it was a safe place and didn't see why there would be any problems with it. I would continue to try and make new and good Facebook friends during that entire semester.

Spring Break Wind Ensemble Tour to Florida.

Once again, I was still having issues with making friends in real life. I really liked a couple of girls that I was going to school with. They were so pretty, and I thought that they seemed nice at least to others. I remember wanting to talk to them so badly. I thought that maybe this would be the year in which I'm able to talk to a girl and get her to go on a date, and maybe possibly date her.

There was a girl in wind ensemble in which I liked as well. Since we would spend a tremendous amount of time together performing and going on tours I thought that I would be able to get to know her. However, my attempts to ask her for coffee were always turned down with her saying some sort of line about being busy or something. The funny thing was that she'd say that she was busy at that time, but then during that time frame I would sometimes see her at the coffee shop on campus grabbing coffee herself.

This year the wind ensemble was scheduled to travel to Florida for the spring tour. Most everyone was excited about this at it met warm southern weather instead of the cold artic weather that we had endured the previous spring tour up in Minnesota and Wisconsin.

In the weeks leading up to spring break I was starting to get a little lonely and depressed. It was really hitting me that I didn't any real friends. My friends were people in which I saw on television such as actors like Cameron Diaz, and they were also people who I would see on the news particularly local news anchors. Up until about this point I was able to deal with it a lot easier but as I began getting older, there was something that set off an alarm in me that was trying to tell me that there's something wrong with me. I just began to become more aware of the situation. I could tell just by observing social interactions just how different mine were from everyone else's. They had to know something I didn't. I would keep on searching as I was still bound and determined to find out exactly what it was that they knew. I needed answers and I needed a solution to my problem immediately.

Meanwhile as we were getting ready to take off for Florida on our spring break tour I was finally asked to be involved with a cousins wedding. I had spent my entire summer sitting around and waiting if I would be asked to be in his wedding or not in some shape or form. I remember getting a phone call from him two days prior to his wedding asking me if I wanted to be in it. Unfortunately, by the time he decided to call and get a hold of me, I had already signed up for wind ensemble and was leaving on the Saturday morning of his wedding. I couldn't do it.

The Saturday in which we were leaving for Florida I had mixed emotions. I loved to travel and was glad we were going somewhere warm, but I was starting to feel overwhelmed by spending large amounts of time with big groups of people. I wasn't sure what was causing it at that point, but I did know that it was uncomfortable. Sometimes when we would perform on these tours I would feel crowed because the venues in which we played in were so small that the ensemble would practically have to sit on top of each other.

The bus ride down to Florida would prove to be a long one. I think we left the school at around 4:00AM on that Saturday morning. I didn't sleep any the night before because I would have had to have driven back over to the school from my house at such an early hour, that I decided it would be best to just not go to sleep and try and stay awake. I often have had this phobia about early morning things. It's a phobia about being late to something if it's going on early in the morning. I don't know why, but I get very anxious the night before and almost drive myself nuts in the head because I'm so busy overanalyzing things and hoping that I won't oversleep and show up late.

The bus was headed for Florida and I will have to say it was one of the more interesting bus rides of my time. The first bus driver was somewhat of a crazy driver. I remember looking up to see him talking on his cell phone, smoking a cigarette, and driving the bus all at the same time. In my mind I was thinking wow, this guy a talented person, then the other thought was, what if he's not a talented person. I wonder what would happen.

Eventually we made it to Florida all in one piece. One of the guys I knew well Paul had to drive the van down that had a trailer full of our equipment on it and he would follow the bus. I remember Paul drove all night on this trip and had some company in the van.

I can't get any girls and he can get two?

I still remember that spring tour like it was yesterday. Some interesting things would happen on that tour and I would end up having an overall good time. While there were still the disappointing social situations, I managed to get the most out of the trip which was a positive thing for me as it was quite possibly the last big positive thing to occur in my life for a couple of years after that.

This guy by the name of Paul had a girl named Abbi that had become fond of him during the fall and spring of 2005-06. They would ride on the van together during this spring tour. Then on top of that there was another girl who just happened to be named Abby who really liked Paul to. This was fascinating to me as I saw Paul becoming quite the ladies' man. I was wondering how he did it? Paul is a great guy and I think he is incredibly nice to his wife now. His current life is Abbi, who is the same Abbi, that I'm talking about here in this story. I was in a room with Paul, Phil, and Justin a few of the guys in which I roomed with on tour and I remember that week being full of "girl talk."

Like they were just talking about girls and their situations
constantly in the room. While, I loved this, I felt a little left
out because I never have had a girl interested in me like
that and I didn't really know a whole lot about girls at all. I
just kind of let what they were saying go in one ear and out
the other. I did this because I knew that if I listened to
them talk about the girls repeatedly it was going to drive
me nuts.

Sometimes when I'm in situations with a group of people in
which they are talking about having successful social lives
I must withdraw from the conversation. Don't get me
wrong, I'm extremely happy for them but when I hear
about how great their social life is and think about how
horrible mine is I immediately tear up and start crying.

During the rest of the tour Paul and Abbi would become
closer to each other. That tour was a lot of fun and I had a
chance to see some awesome things. I remember that I
took my digital camera with me so that I could hopefully
capture some of the scenery. We were down south and
there were hills and mountains. The weather we had was
perfect. It might have rained once that week, but I can't
recall any day being a complete washout.

There were a few nice days in which we would have a half
hour or so to enjoy ourselves and relax and I remember one
place in which there was a huge lake nearby and I thought
it would be a good idea for the group to take a picture
together in front of the lake. I was and still am big on
getting pictures taken whenever I'm with someone. I never
used to know why this was, but I've figured it out over the

past few months.

I want to have pictures taken when I'm in a group because I want something to remember the people by. Since it isn't very often at all that I get the chance to hangout in a group of people, I wanted to have memory of the event. I wanted to be able to see the people in which I considered friends many years from then. In fact, I still have several pictures from way back then and try and look through them quite often.

I also really wanted to have pictures of me taken with a couple of girls. I wanted to have a picture taken with me standing in between two girls. I'd often see pictures of guys on Facebook standing in between two girls and they had their arms around each other and I remember thinking that this guy was the coolest guy in the world. Girls wanted to be in a picture with him. I remember often going around the group during this spring break and trying to ask a girl if we could take a picture together and they acted funny about it. I guess I was doing something wrong by asking them to be in a picture with a guy like me.

I think that instead of coming right out and saying I think you're pretty, would you be in a picture with me, I may have hinted around at it. Maybe that was my mistake. Possibly if I would have just been straight and came out and said, I think you're pretty, would you be so kind as to take a picture with me then possibly they would have said yes. Again, being so socially inexperienced and unaware I didn't have any idea how to ask her so I just kind of hinted at it hoping that they would just give me a chance to take one picture with them.

After trying to get them to take pictures with me and failing, I was able to manage talking Mr. Flanagin into getting a group picture taken in front of the lake. Again, this made for a great background to an incredible picture and I still have the picture of the 2005-2006 Indiana Wesleyan University Wind Ensemble hanging in my room.

Saving the Day So the Musician Could See.

This would be something that would happen that I can say was positive for me as it did give me a sense of accomplishment in a sense. It allowed me to feel good about myself. It was towards the end of the week and we were getting ready to do our last few performances. We were on the bus ride in between one church and heading to another. As we were getting closer to the church we were going to perform at that evening one of the section leaders in the group who played flute lost her eye contact and we couldn't find it.

Jenna is a nice person and she's an amazing musician. The girl can play the flute like I've never heard anyone play it. I often think it's quite unfortunate that she wasn't music major and is not currently performing in the New York Philharmonic, but I know that she's passionate about what she's doing now as she loves kids.

So, everyone on the bus was looking for her eye contact and I being the musician I am was going crazy because not only did Jenna not have an eye contact to see for the rest of the trip, but she didn't have an eye contact to see the music at that night's performance. I'm sure she probably had every piece of music memorized but still it's nice to have the ability to see a passage of music sometimes just to make sure you've got it down.

After several people had spent several minutes looking for her contact and everyone had pretty much given up hope and returned to what they were doing, I remember thinking that I'd try one last place. There were several empty Wal Mart sacks on the floor of the bus since all of us liked to have snacks while on the bus. After looking down and checking through a couple of bags I eventually came to a bag that had a small contact in it. I had saved the day. Jenna could see again, and I was happy. I think she was happy to. She said thank you so much which meant a lot just to hear a girl say thanks or even say hi. I will always remember that day and time as one of the better days in life so far. I was able to help someone out and they were able to see again, and she really appreciated it.

On the way home, we stopped to perform at a church in Alabama. There was a valley right next to the place in which I stayed at that evening and I was amazed at just how wonderful the scenery was. It was great to be able to look out into a valley across the mountains and see for miles. I wouldn't mind living down south someday as I think it could be extremely beautiful and very relaxing. I love the Smokey Mountains and just plain traveling in general. Especially if you can go somewhere to where the weather is half way decent year-round. Sounds perfect to me.

After returning home from our spring tour that year we

only had about a month and a half of school left. Since I had walked out of Ponderosa Steakhouse the previous year, I would have to try and find some sort of a summer job to keep me busy and try to make a little extra money to have. I actively began searching for summer employment.

Meanwhile back at school we were doing some end of the year things in wind ensemble. The honors brass quintet along with the saxophone quartet and various other small ensembles throughout the group had a chamber music series concert right after the spring break. We performed some music that had been composed by a good friend of mine and enjoyed our last official performance together. This was a remarkable experience getting to play with such talented and dedicated musicians.

Finishing up the year would be a bitter sweet experience for me. I'd never finished a complete year of college before and I did manage to pass all my classes. This would be the last semester in which I have been able to complete an entire semester without dropping out of at least a class or two in each semester.

14 TRY AGAIN

The summer of 06 was probably one of the most interesting summers up until this point. However, the summer of 2007 would eventual top it and leave it way behind and in the dust. In late spring of 2006 I decided to apply for a summer job at General Motors. I thought this would be a great opportunity for me to meet some people and make a lot of good money because they paid college kids to come in as summer help and gave them twenty dollars per hour.

In May I had to go and spend one Saturday afternoon up in Fort Wayne to do some testing. They would bring all the college kids in for testing. If we passed the test, then you'd be put into a pool to wait and see how many college kids they needed for the year. I was kind of excited and hoping I would get the job at General Motors. I didn't have anything else going on for the rest of the summer and I thought maybe I could even work second shift which would allow me to sleep in and make even more money.

The Phone Call

One afternoon in early June, I remember getting a phone call. They said that it was General Motors and they were asking me if I would be interested in working at GM for the entire summer. I said of course as I was pumped to make up a lot of money and save it. I thought that maybe I could get myself a nice thing or two at the end of the summer and save the rest to live off for college.

I had never been so excited in my life. Probably because I'd never had the chance to make so much money while I was working. I mean I was going to college, so I could make this kind of money, but to have a chance to just make big money all summer long and bank it was something I would cherish.

Meanwhile in late May I had met a girl on an online dating website from not too far away from here. She went to Indiana Wesleyan University as I would later find out. At first, she was kind of mean and skeptical then she started to really get to know me and thought that possibly we could hangout or I could take her shopping or something to that nature. So, a couple of weeks later we would hangout for the first time. We went up to Fort Wayne and did some looking around and had dinner. I had a great time and I was hoping that she did too. In fact, it seemed as if she did but then later she would kind of blow me off and want nothing to do with me.

When I asked her out again she would say that she couldn't because she didn't want to ever get married or have kids. She told me this but, yet she was on a dating website. This really confused me. So, I just kind of let it go and tried to move on like I always did. Thinking that every girl would hate me for the rest of my life. At least I had the job at General Motors lined up and could make some money and get ahead during the summer of 2006, at least that was the plan.

About four months later I would find out that this girl who had told me she couldn't hang out with me anymore because she didn't want to ever get married or have any kids was engaged to be married. No joke. Just four months after telling me that, she was now ready to get hitched suddenly? "How does this happen?" I asked myself.

So, on June 12th I would report to General Motors for my first day of work. The first two days would be spent training and then on the third day we would go out to our jobs and try to start training on them. Working on the assembly line was one of the coolest things that I've ever had the chance to do in my life. I really enjoyed the pace of things and was able to work on my own and not have to do anything with anyone else, even though it was one huge team. I tended to work better in one on one situation as opposed to working with large groups of people all at once.

I was very nervous during the training sessions though as they were in the mornings and there would be a lot of people all in the same room and even some big shots from the company. I was always afraid that I wouldn't be good enough to do the job that they wanted to do. In any job I've had I've never thought that I would be great at it because I have some sensory issues. The problem is that when they don't know you're having sensory issues, they don't know how to help you. So, since I didn't even know I had Asperger's Syndrome at the time there was no way in which I could get help on any job that I was doing.

We would often get a little break every now and then during the meetings because all we were doing was sitting there and watching videos about the job and people would tense up and get tired, so to keep everyone awake they decided to give us some breaks. During these breaks I noticed that not only were the other people going to the bathroom, but they were also standing around and talking to each other outside of the room. This was interesting to me because I couldn't do this like they were. I immediately felt left out and just wanted to go back into the room and get on with the rest of the class. I wish I knew how to get myself involved in social conversations but it's a huge struggle for me.

After spending the two days of training basically locked inside of a classroom I was ready to get out and start my job. While I was nervous that there was a chance that I wouldn't be able to do it and others would make fun of me, I liked being active more so than sitting in the classroom. I had to be doing something to keep my mind off things and this was the perfect opportunity to do something productive that would keep my mind away from the negative in life and make me some money all at the same time.

They ended up drafting me to work in a section of the facility called "Trim four." This was where much of the detail work was done to the inside of the trucks as they passed down the line. I remember being put into the position of being the person who had to put the middle consul in the truck. Along with this I was supposed to peel off two stickers and place them inside the trucks glove compartment. I had anywhere from thirty to forty-five seconds to accomplish all this which wasn't too bad.

I would however have some trouble with putting the stickers in the glove compartment. This would be like the easiest part of the job and yet I was having trouble with it. I thought I was just stupid, but I couldn't get the stickers to peel off very easily and once I did get them off they were bent, and I had to try and force them to stick to the glove compartment. This is also a job that needs to be neatly done and having Asperger's usually means that you're not the most neatly organized individual.

The reason why General Motors brings in college kids over the summer is because GM full time employees have such amazing benefits that some who have been there for a while may have up to as much as six to eight weeks' vacation in which most people want to use during the summertime. The college kids are just temporary replacements to their full-time employees. I had a guy train me on putting in the middle consul and he was nice. He was probably in his late 40's or early 50's. I remember watching how much time he had to goof around in between jobs. He once told me that if he works an entire shift, he's able to put a seat in the truck in about ten seconds, leaving twenty-thirty-five seconds in between each truck. He told me that he reads the entire USA Today front to back just while sitting on his job. He doesn't even have to read during his breaks. It's crazy how it works but he was such a nice guy and really taught me how to do the job well so that the transition was easy.

Other people couldn't really see me performing my job so even if I was doing something wrong they wouldn't get the chance to laugh at me or make fun of me. This, I was grateful for. My job was easy, and I quickly caught on. Except for the sticker problem this would be a job that I'd become a master at. I got to the point in which I started to look forward to going in to work at around 4:30PM in the afternoon. This was something that I truly enjoyed. There were a few people that I would get to know on this assembly line in which I worked. There was a guy in his thirties and a few others that really seemed to like me and think that I was a good worker. I enjoyed their company and appreciated their thoughts.

Starting a New and Somewhat Bad Habit

As my life was going on and I was still not having any success at all in social relationships and zero success at all with talking to girls I began to brainstorm and try and come up with some reasons. I mainly focused in on the reasons as to why girls didn't like me. I didn't care so much about the guys not liking me and I don't even to this day to tell you the truth. I mean it would be great if they could or would, but it's just there have been guys in my life who have really taken advantage of me and used me as well as physically abused me. This is something that I just can't get over and act like it never happened. There is no trust there for guys. I think it will be a long time before I trust a guy to be a close friend unless he's an older guy who's more like in his late thirties or forties and up.

I thought that maybe my problem with girls was that they thought I was fat and ugly. I couldn't think of any reason at all as to why they wouldn't give me a chance to even get to know them. It had to be me or how fat I was. Since I thought I was very unappealing to girls in the way of looks (being too fat and ugly) I would go down a very dangerous road for a while.

I immediately decided that I was going to do something about the problem. I wasn't even fat really at all as I was only around 166 lbs. at the time and I was 5'11. But it wasn't based off what I thought of myself the decision to start doing some of these things were based off what I thought girls though about me.

I decided to up my number of crunches I was doing per day from 1000 to 2000. I then immediately started walking for one half hour every day. Eventually as I would encounter more situations with girls I would decide that I must not being doing enough, or I must not be trying hard enough. I would up my crunches to 3000 every day and walk the half hour and then start running a half mile every day. I couldn't miss a day of this because I had to lose weight so girls would like me.

On top of all the extra hard working out I was doing I immediately decided that I had to stop eating. Girls hated

me because I was so fat and ugly, so I had to lose some
weight. My goal was to get down to 120 lbs. so that girls
would like me or think I was at least cool to talk to. There
was no way I was going to live my life like this anymore by
sitting around waiting. I had to make a change and become
more attractive to them. Something had to be done.

I started to go through phases in which I would not eat
three or four days straight at a time. I didn't want any part
of having food because I knew food equaled me becoming
fatter and that would mean girls hating me even more than
they did. The goal was to lose fifty pounds and not gain. I
couldn't lose fifty pounds by eating. After going three or
four days in a row without eating there were times when I
became exhausted and a little sick. I thought this was a
normal thing, so I didn't really let it concern me too much.
There was no way I was going to start eating again. I had
this big goal in my head at times that I wasn't going to eat
anything ever again until a girl at least would talk to me for
five minutes.

I didn't even want to look at a plate of food. This is
something that I started in late spring of 2006 and would
continue off and on for about two years of my life. I had
decided that I was going to lose weight and I was going to
get a girlfriend.

Now that I was working at General Motors and was
bringing in a little more money I quickly joined as many
dating websites as possible as I just so desperately wanted
to meet a girl. I joined several of them. I was on them for
about two or three weeks before I would meet a girl. Her

name was April.

As I met April I would begin talking to her at about the same time as my two-week vacation was getting ready to begin. Now I didn't receive a paid vacation from General Motors but being summer help, I did get two full weeks off. General Motors shuts down for the first two weeks of July every year. I wasn't sure what I was going to do with myself for these two weeks. I didn't have any social activities planned because I didn't know anyone really and I just wasn't quite getting it. I was on the outside looking in, which is where I've spent my entire life on the social arena.

Friday, June 29th, 2006 was our last day to work at General Motors before the two-week shutdown. I can remember us getting out a couple of hours early that night since they must completely shut the line down before the company officially goes into shut down mode. So here I was two weeks' vacation and nothing to do.

It was on that following Saturday morning. Saturday, June 30th, 2006 in which I would meet April. April was from Michigan. She lived about four hours north of Fort Wayne, Indiana. She was twenty-four years old at the time and she had just gotten out of a relationship. That last part about her getting out of a relationship met absolutely nothing to me at the time. It wasn't until later when it was too late when I'd begin to understand the significance of that.

April and I immediately began talking and getting to know each other. This was the first time in my life in which I girl wanted to give me any attention. We talked for about three hours on an instant messenger that's associated with a dating website and we seemed to get along, so she gave me her phone number and told me to call her the next day.

I was immediately excited and had high hopes. I had never had any kind of a girlfriend or a kiss at all. I was thinking could this be the first time I get to hold a girl's hand or kiss a girl? I called her up on that Sunday afternoon and talked with her for a couple of hours. She was getting ready to leave town to go on a trip with her church. She was headed off to Oklahoma for a week, but she wanted to meet up for dinner when she got back to Michigan, so I said okay.

It was on the Sunday evening before she left in which we talked on the phone for about ten hours. I had never had any kind of experience with a girl in my life. Not even talking on the phone or texting a girl too often. This was a whole new experience for me, so I wasn't sure what to think of it.

Obviously, I liked having the attention from a girl. After talking on the phone for nine or ten hours on that first evening, she left for Oklahoma but continued to call and text me all day long. That first Monday I bet I had around 200 text messages from her and we talked on the phone that night. At that point and time, I was still loving the attention as I wasn't used to it. So, I was still excited and couldn't wait to meet up. She continued texting me and calling me, I would guess that I would get anywhere from 300-500 texts per day from her and a few phone calls. It was like she really liked me.

I quickly became interested in her sense she was willing to

pay attention to me. She started emailing me these things called E-Cards and sending me random text messages and was great. However, later in that week I noticed something that I think was a red flag but at the time with my social unawareness I had no idea what was going on. I was so caught up in the moment that I probably ignored any red sign that was there.

It was about Thursday of that week when April was still texting me constantly and calling me repeatedly in which I thought it was a little strange and I wasn't sure if I was ready to be texting a girl 500 times per day and calling her 10 or 20 times, but I thought this was normal. On that Thursday night I tried to talk to her about it by telling her I wasn't sure about this and if it was going to work because it just felt kind of weird or awkward. She immediately freaked out and started to beg me to give her more time and another chance. She had been through a lot in the past and she just really liked me she said so I thought okay, we'll try and give her more time and another chance, so I did.

The rest of the weekend continued like the first half of the week. I think she may have tamed her texting down a little bit. That was the first time in my life in which I was ever introduced to texting. I ended up having to go into my cell phone store and getting an upgrade, so I could send and receive all the texts that she was wanting to share.

The rest of that weekend was spent relaxing around the house. I continued my running and my working out with 3000 crunches daily. I was walking a half hour and running a half mile as well. I wanted to be sure that I was in perfect shape for when I met her.

As the weekend went on we would continue to text back and forth quite frequently. Again, thanks to my lack of social awareness and since I'd never even been on a real date with a girl, I would have no idea of what was supposed to be normal or abnormal behavior for a girl in a dating experience.

Finally, after a long-awaited week and a half in which I had to wait and wait for her to come home from Oklahoma she would arrive back to Michigan. She came into town late Sunday and we planned on hanging out on Monday. I was so excited about this because it was going to be my first date ever.

Finally, at the age of twenty-one years old I was going on my first date. Of course, I had to drive nearly four hours to experience my date, but I was about to break the ice and have my first real date with a real woman.

I woke up bright and early on the Monday, July 10th, 2006 and I began to workout. I did my normal routine and then I came back, showered, got in my car and hit the road for Michigan. The ride up to Michigan was a peaceful one as I listened to music. She did call me and text me a few times during the ride up updating me of her day as she had some errands to do in the morning.

Finally, at about 12:00 PM I met up with her. I was quickly amazed and impressed with how beautiful she was. We then sat and talked for a little bit before getting a picnic lunch prepared and heading to the park to enjoy it. The park was amazing as it was a picture-perfect weather day. The temperature was nice, and the sun was shining.

We spent about seven hours together that day before parting ways. Both of us had a good time. We had went to a picnic in the park, a movie, then dinner at Applebee's and finally to get some ice cream. It had been a very busy but productive day.

I left and headed home feeling the greatest that I have ever felt about myself. I had finally experienced somewhat of a successful interaction with a woman. I was excited and nervous all at the same time. I didn't know what to think of this whole girlfriend thing or the possibility of having a girlfriend.

It was decided that we would hangout again on that Friday. It would be such a long week for me as I was even more excited to see her the second time than I was for meeting her the first time. I couldn't wait until Friday. I was so happy. When I arrived home I immediately wanted to start telling everyone about her.

The rest of that week we spent talking on the phone and texting back and forth. We were starting to get comfortable with one another and this was making for a good time. Meanwhile back at home I was continuing with my workout routine and trying to avoid eating as much as possible. Just because I had finally received some attention from a girl, it didn't mean that I could let up. No, I had to work even harder to make sure that I was in shape and she wouldn't think I was fat or ugly.

On Thursday, July 13th of 2006 I thought that I had a wonderful idea pop into my head. I thought that I would make the four-hour drive to Michigan just to drop some flowers on her door step and come home without her even knowing that I was there. So, I got in my car and drove up to Michigan. I had done some research and learned of a few great flower shops around the area so as I got there I immediately started searching for them.

Meanwhile during my entire drive up there she was texting me constantly from work. She had just started a new job and was at training for it. She was apparently bored at the training, so she started texting me. This was cool because I was like thinking to myself "I'm on the way up to drop some flowers off at your doorstep."

I went to the flower shop downtown in the city in which she lived and was able to find a dozen roses. I picked up the dozen roses and went for her place. I left them at the doorstep to her apartment and then I got in my car and proceeded to come home. I thought that just by doing something this simple you could really make a girl's day and make her smile.

About twenty minutes after I'd left her place I got a phone call from her. She said that she came home and was surprised to find some flowers sitting on her doorstep. She read the card and was calling to thank me. See, I think that guys should do little things for girls like this all the time. Why don't they do this? I wonder.

I had arrived back home that evening with enough time left to once again talk with her on the phone and tell her goodnight. Then I proceeded to relax. I watched some television and did a little bit of reading. For the first time in a long time I was feeling happy and wanted to keep it this way.

On Friday, July 14th I went up to Michigan to see her again and spend most of the day with her. We had another picnic in the park and then watched a movie. I helped her with some baking she was doing, and we just hung out and relaxed. It was a wonderful afternoon and I was learning to enjoy myself in a woman's company.

Then I would have to go a week or so without seeing her which wasn't a big deal at the time. It was during this week that I would learn more about her. I had learned that she expected me to take her shopping and buy her expensive gifts. Luckily for me this wasn't going to be a problem at all. Since I was working at General Motors. So, as time went on and we continued to talk on the phone and communicate with text messaging we were drawling closer to meeting again on Saturday, July 22nd, 2006. I was excited, and I had went out and bought her a necklace so that she could have some jewelry to wear.

She had also told me she would like some new clothes to wear. So, I immediately started looking for clothes I could get her. She had a lot of wants and she wanted me to get everything for her and so I was bound and determined to make her happy and very willing to do whatever it was going to take.

Unfortunately, my plans of saving all that money that I was making over the summer at General Motors had quickly gone out the door and I instantly began spending instead of saving. I wanted her to know that I liked her and apparently it was going to take buying her nice gifts and giving her money to show her that I liked her. It was just like the other girls I had met in my past, I had to buy them stuff or give them money just to get them to think about having coffee with me. At least with this girl it would be a little different in that fact that she did hangout with me more than once.

Finally, after a long week of waiting, a week in which saw both her and I go back to work. A week in which I found out that she was expecting me to communicate with her 24/7. She even wanted me to call her at 3AM every morning just to wake her up and talk to her on her way to work. So, I would get home from my job around 1:30AM and then try and force myself to stay awake so I could call and talk to her at 3:00AM.

After a long week, I was done with work. I went home to get a little bit of sleep on that Friday evening before waking up early the next day to travel to Michigan to spend the day with her. The fact that I was dating someone kind of or at least had more than one date with them was an accomplishment that would make me feel extremely good about myself.

I woke up bright and early the next morning ready to go. I did my 3000 crunches, walked a half hour and ran a half mile. I was ready to go and excited to give her all her gifts that I had gotten for her that week. She said that she really loved getting gifts and that was the only way anyone could be her boyfriend is if they kept buying her stuff. I didn't want to screw up or lose her, so I thought the more I buy, the better of a chance I will have at her liking me long term and wanting to date. This was at least the message that she was sending me.

Getting too Excited

At this point, as feel as if it's important for me to touch a little on the subject. For me, whenever something good happens in my life socially there is tendency to grab onto it and want to wrap my arms around it and keep it in my life. This is something that I must continue to work on every day of my life. When something good happens it's okay to get excited about it and feel great about it. However, if you are too obsessively excited about it, there can be some problems. Especially it's another human being. Sometimes excitement scares people off.

This is a lot of the case sometimes for individuals who aren't on the spectrum. You see, neurotypical individuals are so used to getting attention from other individuals that sometimes they become annoyed or bothered with too much attention. NT's already have this awesome network of people set up that includes, friends, co-workers, relatives, other business people. They have so many people in the sea to pick and choose from when they need someone or want someone to talk to that all they need to do is pick up their phone and dial someone's number. There's always someone that wants to talk to them or hangout with them.

For those of us on the spectrum, we don't have anyone

hardly ever pay attention to us. We spend so much of our lives being ignored that when someone finally does decide to try and get to know us we tend to jump on it and want to take it in all at once. While I'm not saying that this is a bad thing at all, and I can completely understand and relate as to why people on the spectrum would do this. I am saying that it is an observation of mine that if you're trying to establish a relationship of any kind with a neurotypical individual, whether it be a friendship with guys, a friendship with girls, or a dating relationship, with a guy or girl, that when the person does show us a little bit of attention that we like and we jump on it too fast and get too overly excited about it we will most likely scare the neurotypical person away who was trying to take time to get to know us and understand us. This is simply because to them this seems creepy. I have often been told by girls that I'm creepy. I have no idea why I am creepy because I certainly don't intend to, but I've learned that it's probably because I come on too strong because of how excited I am, and they are used to guys that play the game of being hard to get.

So, after that much awaited week I was finally on my way up to Michigan to see April. It had been about eight days since we'd seen each other last so I was kind of excited just to see her again. I had planned a rather eventual day around Michigan that I thought she would enjoy, plus I had all these gifts here with me to get to her. I was particularly excited about the necklace in which I was giving her. It was 10 KT Gold. I spent about six-hundred dollars on it and couldn't wait to show it to her and have her try it on.

When I arrived, I was surprised to see that her mom was still at home. I hadn't exactly planned on meeting anyone's parents yet, but she surprised me by introducing her to her mother. Then we sat around a talked for a few minutes and I was able to give her some of her gifts. These gifts were something that I thought she would like very much and think were special. So, I was glad to see the delightful smile on her face when she opened the necklace.

After she had opened all her gifts we then decided to go out for lunch. We spent the day going to lunch, doing some shopping at the mall, going to a movie in the movie theatre, going out to a nice dinner, and then getting some ice cream. The day was most enjoyable and relaxing. I loved the fact that I had someone to spend time with and hangout with for the first time in my life. I enjoyed it so much that I really hated to say goodbye when the day was over.

That day when we were together we had done some talking and it was suggested that we make up a song. A song for us. So, we began listening to some music and we really fell in love with a Stephan Curtis Chapman song called "I Will Be Here." To me the song said so much about how a guy should treat a woman. I liked the song and being a music person, it was kind of important to me that the music be of good quality and taste. This song fit all my requirements and she liked it. So, "I will Be Here" became our song.

That evening after departing Michigan and heading for home, I played the Stephan Curtis Chapman cd all the way home. I was so excited that I even listened to the song over and over. In fact, I don't think I listened to anything else at all on my way home. After getting home I proceeded to upload it to my computer almost immediately. That's how important it was to me. I wanted to get it uploaded.

Later, as time would go by I would even try to memorize all the words to the song. I spent a week just memorizing the song. I thought that it would be a nice gesture if I were to memorize every line to the song and then call her one day and sing it to her on the phone. Or even better, sing it to her in person sometime. Now I wasn't anything close to the world's greatest vocalist, I mean I played trombone. So, singing was a stretch for me, but I wanted to show her how special she was and just how much I cared about her.

I wanted her to know that I was going to go above and beyond to do great things for her to make her happy and feel appreciated. I even wrote her little cards and sent creative messages. Life was great. I was getting to communicate how I felt with a girl and she was getting to feel appreciated. What could be any better?

After spending the whole week practicing the song and going shopping to get her some gifts as well as going about my other daily activities such as working out and working, I was ready for yet another weekend. I was ready to go and hangout with her once again.

It was during this week that I had bought her a couple more outfits and even a pair of earrings. I was so excited. I think part of it was the excitement of just having a girlfriend and someone to buy things for that would make her happy and someone to do nice gestures for that I liked very much.

I was ready to go and on Saturday, July 29th, 2006, I left very early in the morning. I was ready to spend the day with her and show her all these great things. It was another nice day and there was not even a cloud in site. I remember listening to our song all the way back up to Michigan and thinking that it was a special song. To this day I don't listen to the song anymore because of the memories.

I arrived in Michigan and she was ready and looking very gorgeous. We went out about our normal routine. I gave her the gifts and she loved the earrings. It was wonderful. Great things were happening, and I was feeling like I was on top of the world. I couldn't wait to introduce her to my family.

We again went to lunch, then shopping, killed some time at her place in the afternoon, then went to a movie and dinner before heading back to her place again. It was an amazing day and I enjoyed it more than anyone could imagine. Just the fact of being accepted by someone was a huge breakthrough for me and I loved every moment of it and everything about it.

Once again after spending the day with her I was thrilled. I got a hug at the end of the day and life was going so great. I wanted to cherish every moment of this and I took as many pictures as we possibly could. I can't tell you how meaningful it is to have a positive social experience with someone even if it is a very brief one.

The following week continued about like the other weeks had. She kept calling and texting and wanting to talk. I kept talking to her and listening to what she had to say.

Towards the end of the week she had received phone calls for a couple of teaching interviews. She had a bachelor's in elementary education. She finally had a couple of interviews and was excited about that. I remember on a Friday afternoon of August 4th, 2006 she had one of her interviews and I told her to let me know how it went as soon as it was over. Well she happened to call as I was walking into work and I was going through a small area in which I would have no service and she left me a frantic voice message saying that I was supposed to answer the phone when she called and kind of made me feel bad. I thought she was upset that I didn't answer, but I didn't answer because it never rang as I had no service there in that tunnel.

I was so excited for her about having the interview and then having yet another interview lined up on Monday morning that I decided to do something a little extra special. I decided that I would drive up there right after I got off work and surprise her. This was planned out perfectly on my part. At least I thought so at the time. I thought I would leave work, go home and shower, and take all the gifts that I had gotten for her that week and hit the road for Michigan at around 4:00 in the morning on Saturday, August 5th, 2006. So, I did. My goal was to arrive at around 8:00AM or 9:00AM on that Saturday morning and surprise her in some way or another.

During the drive up there, I thought that it might be cool to get her some flowers. I stopped at Wal Mart to buy some flowers as that would be the only place that would be open at that early of an hour in the morning. I had a bunch of daisy's and then I thought that I would stop at McDonalds and get her favorite breakfast meal from there and then take the flowers and the McDonalds breakfast and leave them at her door step. Then I thought I would wait until she woke up and send her a text telling her she better looks outside. I thought that it was going to work out perfect and all. I loved it.

For some reason, I am full of like thousands and thousands of romantic ideas and or nice gestures that one could do for a woman. I've got them all stored within my brain capacity so that I can call one of them into action when I get into a situation in which I think one would be useful.

When April awoke that morning, she began texting me and I explained to her that I thought she should go look out of her front door. So, she did, and what she found were several daisy's spread out surrounding a sack of McDonalds food. It seemed though as if her first thought was what is this? Or why did you do this? Or even, this is weird. I didn't understand why the delay in her response but after several minutes she eventually replied with a "thank you that was really sweet."

I thought that this was sort of strange, but I attributed it to the fact that she was still tired from just waking up. After she got ready and I got over to her place everything was good. We shared some food and talked and then we decided to go about our day. We decided to just take the day as it came to us without really planning too much. We ended up doing a lot of the same things such as lunch, shopping, dinner, and a movie. We also managed to stop at a store in the mall for her to get a manicure. She asked if it was okay if she got one and I told her eyes of course. So, we proceeded about our day after she received the manicure.

That evening back at her place things seemed a little strange to me. She just wasn't very talkative like she usually was. I was exhausted because I hadn't slept all night due to the fact of wanting to surprise her by showing up early in the morning and leaving flowers and food on her doorstep, so I decided to head home as early as possible. I left at around 8:00 that night because I still had a four-hour drive ahead of me. That night while driving home I was doing some more listening to our song. I loved the song and I really liked this girl April. I was so exhausted while driving home though that it was hard to stay awake. I can recall nearly falling asleep while driving home a few times. It was an adventurous drive. April was someone that I liked and wanted to get to know some more. Little did I know that Saturday, August 5th, 2006 would be the last time I would have ever seen her in my life.

It wasn't until later the next day when things started to happen. She told me that she was no longer interested in me and wasn't sure exactly what she had wanted. She wasn't sure of what she wanted in the first place. I had already ordered some more flowers that were going to be delivered to her apartment on that Monday, August 7th, 2006. I wouldn't get a chance to cancel them at all because I was finding all of this out on a Sunday night. I was devastated, and I couldn't understand what I'd done wrong. I wanted to know what happened, but she just said she was no longer interested.

Knowing what I now know today about relationships and girls I now realize that I missed so many red flags and signs about getting involved with someone of this nature. April was 24 years old and she had been dating a guy for about two or three years. In June of 2006 April found out that this guy had basically lied to her about his entire life and existence and about who he was. She was completely devastated, and she ended the engagement.

That all happened in June and I met her on that same June 30th. I knew very well of all this that happened with the last guy. She told me everything, in fact that was one of the reasons why she said she had liked me so much, because I was a sensitive guy who was very willing to listen. She had stated that she'd never had a guy let her complain about a previous relationship for so long.

I am just that kind of guy though. I think girls are amazing sometimes. They deserve that kind of care and compassion. A guy should always listen to them and try and figure out what they need and how to best give them what they need to be happy.

When we first met, and she started texting me and calling me constantly she was quickly ready to move on and get some attention from another guy. It was during this first week in which I met her that something else happened that should have been a red flag. I'm sure that it would have been a red flag to any neurotypical individual who was a guy. Before we even met each other in person after talking on the phone for a little under a week the words "I love you" came out of her mouth. Wow, I'd never heard such amazing words from a woman in my life.

This could have been tragic telling a Neurotypical individual that she loved him before meeting him. Although he most likely would have told her to take a hike because he would have been onto her and have known what was going on. Unfortunately, as someone with Asperger's I'd have no idea what was going on. I thought that this was how dating worked and this was how girls operated. I was just along for the ride and enjoying it.

To summarize here, knowing what I now know, knowing I have Asperger's, having a greater understanding of girls and relationships, and just being more cautious in general, I now know that as soon as she said the words "I love you" before ever meeting me in person that I should have been running away myself, and running fast. Unfortunately, I was unaware of this.

I had a cousin who was trying to explain this concept to me in which I couldn't understand. I was telling him what had happened. I shared with him every little detail of the month or so in which I had known her. My cousin first introduced the term rebound to me. I had no idea what a rebound was. I mean to me a rebound was when someone shot the basketball and missed, and someone grabbed the ball as it came off the rim. That was a rebound to me. I couldn't get grasp as for what the word "rebound" met when dealing with dating and women.

My cousin eventually proceeded to explain to me and try to get me to understand that April had been hurt just right before I met her by another guy and that she was doing what's called a rebound. I had no idea and I still don't understand why someone would do this. I understand that you're hurt but then you're using this guy to try and make you feel better who develops feelings for you and likes you. What did this guy do to you?

The "Aftershock"

I personally have never lived anywhere in the world in which I've had to endure a major earthquake. However, just last spring, in April or May there was an earthquake in which the epicenter occurred in the state of Illinois somewhere. I live in Fort Wayne, IN and was living in on campus housing.

It was in the middle of the night that I awoke to some strange noises. Things were shaking, girls were screaming, and I couldn't figure out why the room around me was moving. It didn't last very long but for a few seconds and I was half asleep, so I didn't really think much about it at the time. However, when I woke up a couple of hours later to begin my day, I was going about my daily walk and jog outside of the dorm rooms when suddenly, another college student holler out of his window at me with "Hey dude, did you feel that earthquake last night?" At first, I was like "What are you talking about but after thinking about it for a few seconds I said yeah, I did."

Then I ran back to my room to turn on the television and try and catch some of the news. Sure, enough the news was reporting that an earthquake had occurred in Illinois. Just a little west of the Indiana/Illinois state line. I couldn't believe that there was an earthquake this close to home. I think I remember one other time in my childhood years in which there was a similar incident.

As is the case with most earthquakes, there would be a few very small aftershocks that occurred throughout the rest of that day. I can remember the day quite clearly. For some reason anytime, there's a big event like this or such as 9/11 I can recall exactly where I was and what I was doing throughout the entire day. It's with such detail to that I'm able to pretty much go through my days without losing any memory.

What happened after April had pretty much picked me up, chewed me up, and then spit me out was what I would compare to an aftershock of a magnitude 7.0 earthquake. I was immediately devastated and distraught and I didn't even nowhere to begin. I needed help immediately. I needed someone to talk to as I just couldn't deal with all the pain.

My body would immediately start shutting down. I'd lose the desire to eat again and become weak. I didn't sleep well at night, but once I did get to sleep I didn't want to get out of bed the next morning. Any motivation that I had in my life was gone within an instant. I needed to pick up the pieces and move on so desperately, but I had no idea how to or where to start. I was a lost young man searching for answers once again. I had thought I had finally solved one of my problems of figuring out how to get a girl to like me but as I was finding out I didn't solve it at all.

I had been crushed and hurt. This girl told me she loved

me, and I fell for it because of how socially naïve and unaware that I was. If only I would have known about the "rebound" thing or what that was all about. If only I could have seen it coming I could have avoided this mess of pain. I had to try and pick up the pieces and move on but for some reason I was just unable to.

That following Monday, August 6th, 2006 I had to go back to work at General Motors in Fort Wayne. I had a hard time with this as I was so depressed that I was unmotivated to do anything at all let alone go spend eight hours in a day at a place where several people would be and work all at the same time. I needed to be by myself and alone, locked in my room where I could cry and talk to my best make-believe friends in the world, Cameron Diaz and Lisa Winter were two of my make-believe friends in which I would try and connect with while I was locking myself in my room.

Yes, even at the age of twenty-one years old, I was secluding myself into my room and turning on the television set to try and talk to or at least listen to Cameron Diaz talk and watch her act, as well as watching Lisa Winter play Basketball.

Obviously, there was a lot more material on television for me to watch Cameron Diaz and try and connect with her, but I did manage to also have some stuff in which I could watch Lisa play basketball.

Thankfully my dad had taped the 1995 IHSAA (Indiana High School Athletic Association) girl's state basketball finals from Market Square Arena in Indianapolis for me. So, I'd always kept that video on file and was able to pull it out and watch Lisa have one of her amazing breakout games of her career against Lake Central in the final game of the year. The Lady Vices would win the state championship that year and I always used to sit in my room and act like I was Fred Fields who was the girls' basketball coach at Huntington North High School.

I quickly re developed the horrible habit of secluding myself from the rest of the world just because I felt so hurt and rejected. The one time in my life in which I really thought that someone was giving me a break or the benefit of the doubt and going to get to know me, it ended up all being a big joke.

Going to work at General Motors became increasingly more difficult. For some reason in which I couldn't figure out, I just didn't want to be there. I was so depressed. I don't think I had ever realized quite how serious my situation was at the time there. It wouldn't be until the following summer to where myself and some of my family would really begin to understand how serious of a problem I was having. For then, I just secluded myself and became even more cautious about people in the real world.

As time went on I didn't get any better. In fact, I would get worse and become more depressed. I was ready to give up on trying for good. I had completely quit eating because I thought I had to be fat and ugly. Why else would she just suddenly up and say you're too nice for me this isn't working out. I knew that she hated me and that I was worthless. This would be the beginning of my fall. From this point on for a couple of years life would be full of many downs and a little up. It was an emotional roller coaster and I was completely drained at times. I needed help but didn't know how to get it and hadn't told anyone yet. I think I was afraid of telling others how I felt out of fear that they would think I was crazy too just like my peers did.

Below is a journal entry that I wrote about four days after April said that I was too nice for her and we were done. This was written on August 10th, 2009.

I don't understand what happened. What did I do wrong this time? I thought that things were going perfect I did whatever she wanted me to whenever she wanted without complaining. I don't get what happened. Why do I feel so hurt right now on the inside? I don't understand why girls hate me. I know that I'm fat and stupid and ugly, but I just don't know why they want to hurt me and be so mean to me. What did I do wrong? I've never hurt them or done anything to them. Why do they hate me? Please please someone tell me what I did wrong? I want to fix it I just want to be the perfect guy for a girl to like. I don't understand why April wouldn't keep getting to know me and give me a chance. She really hurt me. What did I do wrong? I am going to go jump in a cave and never come out. It seems like it would be so much safer in there. The only people that pay attention to me are my imaginary friends that I've created They make me feel good and don't judge me or anything like that at all. I wish that others could be more like them and treat me nice. I want to be like everyone else. I just don't understand what it is that people hate about me. Can you fix it please? Please give me the answers so I can go fix it and be the perfectly cool person everyone wants to hang out with. I r want to be someone else because being Travis isn't working for me. Lisa and Cameron are the only two people in my life that treat me nice and give me a chance. They're on television though and I wish so much that they could be real. Those are the type of people that I want to have around me. Because they don't talk about me or make fun of me. Or steal things from me. They are just cool people with a great personality. I wish more than anything that I could meet them. Please someone take me there and let me meet them. Just let the pain go away. I'm tired of it hurting and want it to leave me. Leave me far alone and never come back. Please go away.

I want life to go on, but you won't leave me be. Please pain go away and never come back. Why do you stay here with me? I want real friends with real feelings and there is none like that here. They are in Hollywood and other various places and I cannot get to them. Please pain, go away and don't ever come back. I need hope, happiness, and peace so why are you still here. I don't know what to do next as I feel I'm about done trying and out of time. Please give me hope and courage to keep on fighting. Where has the happiness gone? It's no longer here. Please come back and never go away. Pain go away, happiness come back and let's never lose each other again. I want a new life, with real friends, and I want to be cool and want everyone to like me and be my friend, please give me that, if not I don't know if I will stay.

I wanted to move on with my life and maybe even start a

new life. I hadn't ever felt any pain like this before in my entire life. As the weeks went on and it became time to go back to school at Indiana Wesleyan I was starting to dread going work more and more. As they found out that I was going to be quitting and going back to school instead of staying there to work full time they started to put me in different areas and tried to make me do jobs I didn't know how to do. I couldn't handle this at this time with all the emotional stress that I was going through. I needed a break and I needed out. It was on the last Friday in August, the 25th that I was put on a job that I really didn't know how to do, and I couldn't figure it out. As time went on I started to get made fun of and teased and I couldn't take it. During one of our breaks I just kept right on walking out the door and never came back. I was done, and I couldn't take any more pain from people. I needed to be alone.

I spent the last week before school started at home pretty much keeping myself locked up in my room except for going out to walk and run. I didn't want to eat family meals and I didn't really have the desire to interact with anyone at all after all the pain that I'd just been through. For a while that summer I was really looking forward to going back to school, but after this event happened it was kind of like, why bother? I was getting sick and tired of the same old story. I try to make a friend or girlfriend and then I fail miserably only to have my heart ripped out, cut into pieces and then sewed back in.

I just didn't know that I really wanted to feel this way at all anymore. I was tired and hurt as well as stressed out and here came another semester in school in which I was going to be taking harder classes than I had to the year before.

15 THE REBOUND

As the summer was ending I quickly realized that it was time for me to start thinking about going back to school. This was not something I was looking forward to now after experiencing what I had over the summer, but I knew it was a must and I certainly had to find something to keep myself busy and occupy my mind.

I was glad to be back in Marion and on campus. There was a brand-new renovation to the student center on campus that would be opening this year. Indiana Wesleyan University had always had some of the nicest facilities around. They always seem to be building something new. I guess that's one of the reasons as to why it costs so much to go to a private school.

I can remember going over to visit campus about three days early before classes were to start just to see some familiar faces. At that point I was really struggling and feeling worthless and miserable. Just to find someone to talk to would provide a huge relief for me. At that point and time, it didn't matter what we talked about so much, it was just the fact that someone was there to listen.

It was while visiting campus within the last weekend before classes were to start that I would run into someone I'd known from when I did some teaching with a local high school marching band. This had been a girl in which would have gotten into an incident with the high school band director that I was helping that year. This situation would be extremely uncomfortable. This girl tried to act like she was my best friend. I hadn't seen her in about five or six months and first thing that happens is she runs up to me and hugs me. Most of the time I like hugs but sometimes if it were to be someone I didn't know very well it would make me uncomfortable.

Since this girl was in the process of accusing the band director I knew and liked of doing something inappropriate it was very uncomfortable for me to be in a situation where I had to talk to her. There were just so many things happening in my life at that time. I was completely devastated about not only the experience I'd had over the summer with April but also the fact that my friend was being accused of something inappropriate. I wanted it to all be a lie and I often wished I could have retreated to the make-believe world to where it wouldn't be such a reality.

As it became time for me to start classes on the Tuesday after Labor Day I was still a mess. I was able to be a little bit hopeful of the fact that maybe something positive would come out of it and I would be able to talk to someone about it and have them understand me and possibly even want to be my friend. For the longest time in my life I was able to hold onto just the slightest glimpse of hope, however as time went on this semester any hope that I had would slowly diminish into being completely hopeless and suffering.

Again, I would like to stress that I believe that coping with rejection and handle it is something that can be very difficult for someone on the spectrum to do. I really believe that people on the spectrum tend to focus in on the rejection so much to the point to where it can really drive them insane. They need to have someone they can trust to talk to about how their feeling or even simply a journal to write in so that they can at least communicate how they feel in some way. I think it's extremely beneficial if someone on the spectrum has a journal and can write in it whenever they feel the need to get something off their chest.

Keeping a journal is going to allow them to voice themselves to someone. Even if no one were to ever read it just the fact that they were able to communicate their feelings to someone (even if it's just someone as simple as a piece of paper) will go along wells in the recovery and coping process for them. I can't tell you how many times I've felt so depressed and rejected that I wanted to hurt myself that I was able to just go to my journal and start writing. Once I started writing it felt like I was able to tell someone something that was bothering me and get it off my chest. While this is no miracle cure and isn't going to make all the pain go away overnight, I do believe that it can go a long way towards helping someone on the spectrum cope.

After trying to get everything in order and get my classes situated and figuring out what day I had what and when I was going to study I was able to calm down a little as far as anxiety, but the depression just wasn't going away. I didn't know what to do. I had been on this path for about four or five weeks now and the pain wasn't getting much better. It was magnifying at times and seeming as if it was worse. I couldn't even function sometimes due to the intensity of the emotional pain. It was completely interfering with my abilities to do my studies as well as anything else I wanted to do. The depression that was seeking in due to being rejected so much was un real and it was quickly destroying my life.

As the semester began I had many obligations. The first of course was to my studies. Then I also had the obligation of playing in as many ensembles as I could, so I could help the music department and enjoy my life. Then there was also the issue of the fact that I needed income. I needed to have money to pay some bills as well as to provide for gas to get back and forth to school. No gas, no school. I had to get some sort of a job and it didn't have to be a high paying job, but it had to be a job in which I could do, and I knew from going through what I went through in the summer and still feeling the amount of pain that I was having that doing any kind of a job that was going to require a significant amount of concentration probably wouldn't be a good idea for me. I had to find something simple, something I could do with ease, and that I was good at.

Eventually after quite a bit of searching I was able to find a nice little job here in the music department on campus. It was a job in which I received through the school. In the United States of America, the federal government has created what they call the "Federal Work Study" program. They created this for students that are going to college. Students enrolled in college courses may obtain a campus job and receive extra financial aid for that job. Depending on the amount of need that the student has the amount in which one would be eligible to receive may vary greatly.

This would prove to be the perfect job for me at this time in my life. I obviously had very poor social skills and so whenever I was forced to work with other people my working skills suffered due to my poor social skills. This was a job in which I would be allowed to conduct my job alone without anyone else being around. I had no other peers involved with me as I was doing mostly work with computers or filing papers. This was something that I could handle even with all the stress and pressure I was under.

I really thought I had found a job in which I would be able to handle with ease with there being no other students or peers around to cause social interference. Again, as I've stated earlier in the book, there is one time in an individual with autism or Asperger's life in which they can enjoy life without any type of a social impairment interfering and this is when they are alone. When they are alone there is no socializing to be done and life becomes much simpler. I believe that this is the key reason as to why people on the spectrum like to be left alone to do their own thing at times.

I don't think they're trying to be rude or unsociable by

doing this. You must put yourself in our shoes, just like we must try and put ourselves in yours. It's easy to assume about someone by judging something that they do, but often what we are forgetting when we make that assumption of someone is that there is probably a good reason as to why they are acting the way they are. It's important that all individuals both on and off the spectrum keep an open mind to each other's feelings and ways of behavior. Let's stop and think before we ridicule someone about a behavior because we really don't know or understand the situation they are in that may be causing them to have that behavior.

Meanwhile the amazing job in which I had secured was proving to be a lot harder for me than I originally thought it would. I thought that because there would be no one else around to tease me or bully me that it would make working a lot less stressful and more enjoyable. But to my disbelief it didn't really help a whole lot. It created a lot more anxiety and caused me to become quite depressed. When I was sitting inside working all alone on some things I was anxious. Because I was sitting inside working while there were thousands of other students running around the university hanging out with each other. These other students were out playing basketball, volleyball, going to lunch or dinner with each other, and getting coffee at McConn which the on-campus coffee shop at Indiana Wesleyan University was. But the point here is that these other students were out running around everywhere and hanging out with one another and it was something in which I couldn't do and wanted to so bad. This caused me to think about it a lot while I was trying to work, and I'd become more and more anxious and less able to concentrate on the important tasks at hand.

It was so bad that I was so anxious that I would just stress out and shut down. I had to get up and walk around every ten minutes or so as I just couldn't sit still. I had to go outside and see what the other students were doing and see if I could become involved in whatever activity they had going on at the time. I really wanted to be included and I never really was. I just couldn't handle it anymore. Going to school and work was so stressful mostly due to the amount of anxiety and depression that was being caused by my poor social skills.

As time went on, I was beginning to realize more and more that something was wrong with me. That would continue to depress me even more. I was searching for answers and had no idea where to start. I couldn't figure it out. I was lost in a world in which I didn't even exist.

Lost in the World that Didn't Exist

There have been many times in my life in which I have felt out of place. A great deal of the time in my life has been spent feeling like I was lost or out of place. There's been times when I've felt as if I was from a different world or belonged in a completely different place. I never quite had a full understanding as to why I wasn't accepted here in this world by my peers nor did I know where I was supposed to be.

I can say that there were times in my life in which I've just felt completely unwanted and wondered if anyone would even notice if I were to kill myself and not here on this earth any longer. In a sense I feel as if I am lost in a world. I'm lost in what is called the "real world." I don't fit in this real world and I can't make connections here or develop friendships. I can't maintain a job here because of the situations that occur for me once I'm in the job. Interviewing for a job is extremely challenging for me. It's hard to make eye contact with anyone let alone someone of importance who is going to be deciding if you're the right person for the job in which they have available.

Even when I have been lucky to somehow impress the interviewer and obtain a job it's been extremely difficult for me to keep it due to the amount of bullying and teasing that goes on at these work places. If bullying and teasing could just be eliminated from the world, then we would all have a much more happy and safe place to live in.

I often wonder to myself how this whole bullying and teasing thing got started. I think back and wonder who was the first person in the world to officially bully or tease someone? If I knew who it was I would want to write them a letter or talk to them in person and let them know what they did was wrong and make them aware of how much pain that they've caused the entire world.

It's almost as if I'm lost within a world in which doesn't even exist for me. While I am very much a part of the real world and I very much try to be to the best of my ability, it's like no matter how hard I try, I won't ever be found within the real world. I could sit here and fight and fight and fight and plead for acceptance into the real world but as of today it's just simply not happened. It's something that I will have to continue to work towards for the rest of my life.

Since I've been unable to be successful at being discovered or found in the real social world, I've created my own little make believe social world. As I've talked about before, many of us individuals who have Asperger's syndrome as well as autism often retreat to our own little world where we can fee accepted and safe.

It is here in this make-believe world in which I've created that I don't have to worry about the guy who tells me he'll allow me to be friends with him if I'll pay him a certain amount of money each month or each time we hangout. I don't have to worry about that beautiful girl in which I like so much and think so much of telling me that she'll have coffee with me if I'll buy her the Television of her dreams or even worse the car of her dreams. I don't have to worry about the class bully pushing me around at school. I don't have to worry about being forced to be tied up to a tree and have punches thrown at me and baseball bats swung at me to pass the group initiation process to become someone's friends or become part of a group. My group is created in my head and they are all people in which don't really interact with me but at the same time they do.

While the people in which I interact with in this world that is safe aren't necessarily make believe or imaginary as they are real life people. One of which is actress Cameron Diaz and the other is my favorite women's basketball player in the whole world, in Lisa Winter. They are imaginary in a sense that I don't ever get to see them in real life or talk to them in person. I get to watch Cameron act in movies such as "Head Above Water" "There's Something About Mary" "Shrek" and of course the infamous "Charlie's Angels" both I and II. I've got all her movies and I really know a lot about her and I do think she's an incredible person.

Then there's Lisa Winter. Lisa a 1996 graduate of Huntington North High School, a school in which I would graduate from eight years later. If a child can have a role model at the age of nine, ten, and eleven, which I really believe they can, then I would have to say that Lisa Winter was the most influential person in my life. I often wonder if people at the young age of seventeen or eighteen which Lisa was at the time in which I was watching her take the state and the nation by storm in the mid 90's know or understand just how much of an influence they can have on someone's life. Now I'm sure that she probably would have never dreamed that she'd have such an influence on a little boy's life as most boys probably think that girls' basketball players shouldn't be playing basketball or that they aren't good. I've often been asked by so many people why I like women's basketball better than men's and it's just one of those things in which I don't see a problem with, but I've been made fun of for it time and time again.

I can attribute the fact that I like girls or women's basketball more so than boys or men's basketball to several things. One of the biggest I think is the fact that I've always been bullied or pushed around by guys. This has really bothered me. A lot of the bullying has involved physical abuse and has led to a tremendous amount of pain.

I don't really feel safe around other guys as I know that I'm generally always going to be put into a situation in which I get taken advantage of, bullied, made fun of, or physically hurt by them.

The game of basketball is kind of similar in such was that it's just a natural thing for men to be more aggressive than women. Men are darn right brutal and men have turned what was the game of basketball or intended to be the game of basketball into some sort of barnyard rough housing game in which mean jump all over each other, push each other, and do all kinds of things that shouldn't be allowed in the game of basketball. Men have basically changed the rule book of the game and ruined its reputation in my opinion. Have you ever noticed that in the NBA guys can take three to four steps without getting called for a travel? This wasn't the case back in the 1980's and before when Larry Bird and Magic Johnson were playing. Back then basketball was still what it was intended to be. How good you were being based on how high you could jump or how good of a slam dunker you were, how good you were being based on how good of a shooter you were and how good of a defensive specialist you were.

Basketball was originally invented to be a non-contact sport. Twenty to thirty years ago there would be no such thing as even touching another guy on the arm. Today the game has been turned into a barn yard brawl. It's almost been turned into a wrestling match instead of a basketball game. This is something that I think the NBA should address as soon as possible. This is also what life has turned into for many people unfortunately.

Just last night, June 14th, 2009 I was watching game five of the 2009 NBA finals. What I was watching wasn't a basketball game? What I was watching was a wrestling match as it appeared to me at times. I mean you would have guys going up for rebounds and getting pushed out from underneath the basket without a whistle even blowing. This is not a knock on anyone from the Los Angeles Lakers or Orlando Magic as both teams had outstanding seasons and I still enjoy watching men's basketball but it's just not the same as watching women's. For some reason the game's been turned into a wrestling match by guy's. It's just something that bothers me. I'm sure that it has a lot to do with the fact that I've always been bullied by other guys and pushed around. But when I'm watching a men's basketball game I start to have flashbacks to times when I was hit or punched in the face or chest, or pretty much wherever you could imagine. It's uncomfortable for me at times when a men's basketball game gets a little too rough and violent. I feel like I need to escape from that situation immediately.

Meanwhile the women's game is a lot calmer and played by the rules in which basketball was intended to be played. I don't think I've seen too many women's games in which a woman has gotten away with taking three to four steps without a whistle blowing. I don't think I've ever seen a woman literally throw someone else out of the lane to grab a rebound without the whistle blowing and them getting called for a foul. The women's game just seems a lot more played by the rules to me and it's also more competitive in my opinion. For some reason, I'm just not very find of other guys. I know it must be because of the way in which

I've been hurt and abused by other guys in my past but it's just that guys and girls approach the game of basketball differently. Guys approach the game of basketball in ways in which I don't and can't understand.

To me it seems as if guys are in it for themselves sometimes. The guys are out for the individual stardom and don't care anything about team recognition or being a part of a team. It seems like guys get in to this big hot dog, I can show off and impress your mode. But that's simply just not basketball at all. But the problem in lies here because most of the world sees something like these guys showing off and trying to draw attention to themselves as entertainment. You see, basketball is no longer about a competition between two teams. It's a competition between twenty-four players to see who can provide the most highlights. This has happened because our society values this as entertaining. It's almost like they go to basketball games now a day to see a real-life television drama series.

Basketball wasn't invented to be an entertaining drama television series however, basketball was intended to be a competition between two teams, to see who was better on that day. Nowhere does it say anything in the rule book about individuals showing off and becoming super stars that make millions of dollars that so many kids look up to. This has been done by society and men. It's no longer just a basketball game, it's a form of entertainment and a way of making money.

Women have a better understanding of the game and the

way it was intended to be played. I believe that the women's game is a lot more interesting than the men's because there is a team competition going on to see who the best team is. There isn't an individual competition going on between a bunch of men trying to prove themselves to the world that they are the best team. The guy's game has become an individual sport as to where the women's game is still a team sport. The ladies have stayed with the rulebook while managing to entertain because they are doing what Dr. Naismith wanted them to.

For some reason, I've always felt safer around girls and women. I feel like my physical safety is in better hands. I think a lot of it has to do with the motherly type figure that they present. I don't know but I long for connection with a lot of girls and women. I am just scared of guys and fear for my life at times when I'm around them. When you've been put in situations in which you've been physically abused repeatedly, taken advantage of, bullied and miss led on things by other guys who just thought it was cool make you feel bad and hurt you, your trust goes out the door and you really must work to trust again.

Guys have equaled a lot of emotional and physical pain for me in my lifetime. From getting told I'm a "stupid piece of shit." To being tied to a tree and having some guys swing a baseball bat at me, I haven't exactly had too many great experiences with guys in my life. I just wish that the pain could go away and maybe I could trust a guy again, but I think that's going to be awhile before I trust a guy who's my age.

Women are just much more "soft." They don't try and act like a macho animal which at times I think it seems as if most guys do. They're much more enjoyable and pleasant to be around as I can tell that they aren't out to physically hurt me in anyway. Again, I think it goes back to the whole sad and hurting boy looking for comfort from the mother. There's a lot to be said for this scenario.

Meanwhile as the fall semester was getting ready to start we had a picnic gathering for the Indiana Wesleyan University Wind Ensemble. The gathering is something that we did at the beginning of the year. We went over to the director's home and had a huge picnic and meeting in which we would all get a chance to introduce ourselves to the group and make some connections. I think this was especially good for new kids that were coming into the group not knowing anyone yet. It would give them a chance to make some connections before the first day of classes started.

Even for someone like me this was a rather useful event. However, I would be forced to try and socialize with people that I didn't know to well as there were some new people in the group. Again, even at a gathering like this it was like the gathering was in some other different world in which I was unfamiliar with and had no idea what was going on. I spent much of the time desperately searching for my own world with people in it that were much like me. This kind of world is something that's very difficult to find for me.

16 LOST

September of 2006 was finally here. I had been struggling with a lot of emotional pain for about a month now, but I was finally going to get a chance to go back to school and get away from the pain. Within the first couple of days of coming back I was able to make myself busy with preparing audition material for ensembles as well as trying to find and get used to all my new classes.

Indiana Wesleyan University was a much more user-friendly campus to me because it was a lot smaller than Indiana University in Bloomington. Indiana University in Bloomington had around 60,000 students on campus at any given time throughout the fall and spring semesters. Indiana Wesleyan didn't have more than 4000-5000 students on campus at any point and time throughout the fall and spring semesters. This made for a much friendlier walking commute to and from classes for me.

I know longer had to try and squeeze in between people to and from wherever I was going. Therefore, there was little or no chance at all that I would slip, trip, of fall due to losing my balance. I sometimes have a difficult time walking in a straight line due to my sensory issues associated with Asperger's. Sometimes I will stagger back and forth a little bit and not even realize that I'm doing it and I may accidentally bump into someone. Whenever I do this I immediately try and apologize to the person, but they still give me some of the dirtiest and meanest looks. I don't do it on purpose.

When a situation like this happens sometimes I just wish that the person on the other end of things could just try and have an open mind and understand what's going on here. But because most people who aren't on the spectrum or neurotypicals aren't educated well enough they tend to have a difficult time comprehending how someone can accidentally do something due to circumstances that are out of his or her control. They just jump to conclusions and assume that the person is being a jerk on purpose and they are ready to call him out for it. They don't think that maybe this guy just has bad balance or something and he couldn't help but run into people.

This all goes back to my visibly/invisibility theory. This is a rather complex thing that I've come up with. I just had the pleasure of writing an article about this the other day. You see, it is said that Asperger's syndrome is an invisible disability. This means that it's a disability that doesn't show up on the outside. No one's going to be able to recognize the fact that I have Asperger's syndrome without talking to me or taking more than a few minutes to get to know me.

I was having a conversation with a group of people the other day, and I asked them to tell me the first five traits or characteristics that came to mind when they looked at me. I heard all kinds of things from funny, intelligent, ambitious, and motivated, but the two words that I didn't hear were "Autism" or "Asperger's Syndrome." This didn't surprise me at all because I'm so used to this. Since getting my diagnosis I've felt comfortable enough with disclosing it to a few people who have been patient with me and allowed me a chance to try and get to know them. When I disclosed my diagnosis to them, not only did they not have the slightest clue as to what it was, but they had no idea I had it and couldn't believe it.

Now when I speak at events I usually open with asking for five or ten volunteers to tell me the first quality or characteristic that comes to their mind when they first look at me. I open with this to prove a point. The point is that Asperger's is invisibly visible. Meaning it's very invisible when you're first getting to know someone, but it becomes extremely visible after the getting to know you process begins.

Today it is my goal to work on helping both the autistic world and the neurotypical world compromise on these issues and come together as one. I would like to see Asperger's continue to be an invisible disability because I believe that disability is one word that it is not. However, what I would like to see is that Asperger's becomes a more visible characteristic in the individual. SO, to sum this up. What I am hoping for is that Asperger's does become more visible to the world and recognizable, however, I'm hoping it becomes more visible in the form of a personality trait as opposed to being labeled as a disability.

We also must take care of this bullying thing that's going on in our schools across the country. I know that my self-esteem was a lot lower as an adult since I was constantly bullied and picked on while going throughout my school years. If I could have just been left alone and not been made fun of I think I would have felt a lot better about myself as a young adult.

Therefore, it's important that we get a message to kids both on and off the spectrum at an early age. We must promote an anti-bullying message that teaches kids that it's not okay to bully someone else or push them around. You see, I believe that a lot of younger kids just don't realize the significance of the effects that can last for a lifetime on someone in which they are bullying or pushing around. We must educate them on this entire subject from an early age, but it must be done in a fun and safe way.

Trying hard to make another connection with a girl.

At the beginning of the school year in the fall of 2006 there was a girl who played the piano who was a freshman and just arriving at Indiana Wesleyan University. She was extremely beautiful and had all the markings of an amazing musician with lots of talent. I knew that she was very good at piano as well as very smart in all academic areas. She was an amazing and wonderful young woman. I wanted to get to know her so bad, so I tried.

It was at a music major picnic/gathering at the end of the

first week of school that I would try and get to know her. I
remember asking her what she was doing that weekend and
then when she said she didn't know or hadn't planned
anything, yet I asked her if we could go on a date. She
looked at me like I had just ruined her day or shocked her
to death and then she was telling other people that I had
asked her on date and it seemed like before I knew it I had
a crowd of people laughing at me and pointing. I was the
joke of the evening and I didn't understand why? I didn't
realize what I had done wrong and then they just all started
making fun of me.

These were all great Christian young men and women who
went to school at Indiana Wesleyan University and they
just started making fun of me because I liked a girl. Well I
think they were trying to tell me to go away but they didn't
want to come out and tell me, probably due to not wanting
to hurt my feelings or whatever so I think they decided to
just laugh at me to make me feel bad so eventually I'd go
away.

That evening after having to experience being put in that
embarrassing situation I immediately took off and started to
drive home. I had tears coming down my face like they
were being let out of a fountain. I cried all the way home.
Once I got home I was going to be secluding myself into
my bedroom and trying to connect with my friends in the
make-believe world yet again. They seemed to always be
there for me when I needed them to be. Thanks Cameron
and Lisa. They probably helped to save my life at times
when I wanted to kill myself when I was just going through
such a hard time and couldn't handle any more pain. I was

able to find some relief in watching them on television and connecting with them.

Once again, I would get sent on a detour into my own little world. I couldn't figure out why this kept happening to me, but I did know that it was a safe place for me to be in and I didn't want to come out at times because I just wanted to feel safe and secure. It was like having a security blanket over you I which no one could harm you. It was very snuggly and comfortable so why come out?

During the entire fall semester of 2006 at Indiana Wesleyan I struggled with many things including academics. It seems kind of odd but when one little thing is off in your body it can have a huge impact on your entire life. Just the fact that you're depressed can totally impact all your daily interactions. My advice to anyone now is if you're feeling the slightest bit of depression make sure you talk to someone about it. I you bottle it all in and keep it on the inside it's only going to get worse, magnify, and intensify until it forces you to explode. So, to anyone who may be on the autism spectrum out there, please talk to people when you're feeling down on yourself.

As we got into the middle of October I would begin crying nearly every day. No one knew what was wrong with me as they all (including my family) just thought I was crazy. I was crying when I woke up, crying in the shower, crying on the drive to and from school, and then crying some more at night when I came home. I couldn't shake the crying and I was starting to wonder why I was alive.

As time went on classes would become increasingly more

difficult and I didn't really have the desire to socialize with anyone at all. I started to lose some desire to even try at social situations. I had lost any confidence in which I had which was already very low. I just couldn't shake all the negative thoughts and feelings and I was seeking help in any way that I could get it.

During this same time the Indiana Wesleyan University Wind Ensemble was slated to go on a couple of fall tours. I remember that I was having a really difficult time and my mother was scared that I was going to hurt myself and asked that the band director kind of kept an eye on me as we were touring. I just wasn't right. I had been hurting for too long and it was starting to have permanent effects on me.

I remember that when we were on the first tour of the year, I just sat on the bus alone and stared out the window. I'd developed a blank stare and I didn't want to really look at anyone. I felt that if I looked at them I was going to get hurt emotionally. I thought that I wasn't good enough for anyone anymore and that the only reason I was even there was because they thought I could play trombone well.

I was just a mess on the trip and people knew it. I sat in the group during the Sunday morning rehearsal and then again when we were at church and tears were just running down my face. I knew I had a problem but at that time I still hadn't heard about Asperger's syndrome. I was sad and lonely, but no one knew why.

After a few weeks of moping around, not wanting to get out of bed, crying constantly, not wanting to eat, and not being able to concentrate on my academics at all, I decided that I needed help. I quickly began searching for ways in which I could get the help I needed. Luckily for me, there was a counseling center on Indiana Wesleyan University's campus. As soon as I found that out I quickly began researching how to get in contact with them and become a part of their program. I wanted counseling. I was able to sign up with Mr. Herr and we immediately began talking about what I was going through. I kept struggling and I didn't know why. I told him about not being able to talk to anyone really, told him I just felt out of place and he was as puzzled as I was.

I went into see the counselor thinking he was going to be the person I've been waiting for my entire life. I was thinking that I'd go in there for an hour and come out with all the answers to all my problems. I thought he was going to be like a super man who could fix any problem that I was having. All I had to do was open to him and tell him what was going on and surely this man would have answers right?

Well, unfortunately it just doesn't quite work like that. Counselors don't just have that super human power that we all want and desire. With anything in life that involves a problem there is a root to the problem in which we must find. This can take some time and it certainly takes more than one counseling session that lasts for an hour.

We talked a lot about social things because this is obviously what I was having the trouble with. One of the main reasons I went to this person was because of my band director, Mr. Michael Flanagin highly recommended him and said that he was great in working with students. I'd never thought about doing any kind of counseling like this before in my life. I just knew that I had no choice but to try and use every available resource that I had to try and find out what the root of my problems were. To me, at that time, the root of my problem was the fact that I was fat and ugly and girls hated me.

The counseling I received from the alters gate center at Indiana Wesleyan University wasn't really that beneficial for me at this time. It did help just to have someone listen to what I had to say, but at this point what I was telling them was that I was depressed, and everyone hated me. I'm sure that everyone involved in my life just that that I was blowing this entire problem way out of proportion.

Again, I can't tell you how many times I've had other people my age tells me that I'm over reacting, and things can't be that bad. They're like, "you're just having a bad day" or it can't be that bad, no one hates you. The problem here is that again, Asperger's Syndrome is such an invisible disability that they can't see or recognize all that emotional pain you're going through. They don't see anything outside of their social bubble so unfortunately since I didn't have the necessary social skills to get inside of their social bubble they didn't see me, much less they didn't see me having a problem at all.

After going to a few counseling sessions on campus there I felt a little better for a brief period. I was able to push myself to get through the rest of the fall semester of 2006.

It wasn't easy, and I had to withdraw from one class because I wasn't able to focus on balancing all four of my classes together at once along with everything else that was going on. I wasn't happy at Indiana Wesleyan and I thought it was because everyone hated me and if I went somewhere else to get away then I may have a chance at developing real friendships with real people.

It was at this point that I would begin looking to make another change in my life. I was still convinced that it was something to do with the environment that I was in that was causing me all these problems. I had convinced myself that all the pain that I was experiencing was because of where I was going to school and if I could just get away and attend a different university then maybe the pain would go away. Maybe, I'd be more accepted. I was searching for answers.

When I was thinking about other places in which I could go to college I immediately thought about Indiana Purdue University Fort Wayne. IPFW is a great school and it's close to home which would again be convenient because I would have to commute back and forth yet again due to my bedwetting problems. In the middle of December, I decided that I was going to try IPFW. Someone had put a thought in my head that the reason that girls at Indiana Wesleyan didn't like me was since I wasn't rich and had very little money. They told me that students that go to Indiana Wesleyan all come from rich family's and I didn't stand a chance with these girls. That person also told me that girls that go to public universities are friendlier and not as stuck on themselves as the ones that go to private universities.

Let me just say, "This isn't true at all." In fact, I would say I've been treated quite a bit worse here at the public university than I ever was by anyone in a private setting. I had a hard time at Indiana Wesleyan because I appeared to be strange, psycho, and creepy to them. I appeared this way simply because they didn't know that I had Asperger's Syndrome. How could they, when I didn't have any idea that I had it myself.

I think there were times while at the school in Fort Wayne where I was taken advantage of by people who didn't even realize they were taking advantage of me. People would sometimes invite me to hangout and then vanish and not be where they were supposed to meet me at. There were a few instances to where I found out that they were doing this on purpose. I tried to just let things like that go at this point because I was so used to it, but I can recall one evening in April of 2007 that really bothered me.

I had met this girl on Facebook who went to school at the same place that I did. After talking for a couple of weeks she told me to come over to her place, so I made the half hour drive down to her place. Then when I got there to hang out with her the place she said to go wasn't the right place. I called her, and she was on the phone saying well go knock at this door and go knock at that door. Basically, I played a game of tag with knocking on every which door I could. I kept holding out positive beliefs that the next door I knocked on the girl I had been talking to was going to answer. That was never the case.

The rest of this semester at the university in Fort Wayne

was spent trying to fit in. I was trying to be like everyone else no matter what it took. My cod characteristics took over though. I started becoming more obsessed with working out and walked and ran farther and farther each day.

By the end of the semester I was at another low point and fighting to stay alive. I couldn't take too much more pain. Late in the semester I met a girl who would play a huge influence in my life. K was a nineteen-year-old college student who had a 3-year-old child. She would be the first girl to really try to help me out instead of make fun of me.

I also met K on Facebook as this had become the way for me to meet people since I would always get rejected in person. I was afraid to try to talk to anyone in person. K ended up giving me her number and meeting up with me. I was so excited. I bought her some flowers and took her to a Komets hockey game. She seemed to enjoy it a lot. We even held hands at the hockey game. Throughout the course of the next week or two I would try and get to know her. For some reason the positive attention I was getting from her made me want even more. So, I kept calling and texting her.

Eventually she didn't respond and asked me to leave her alone too. I thought oh no! I had messed up again. After allowing her to cool off for a couple of weeks though she finally answered a text and agreed to hang out with me again. This night was in late May of 2007 and to this day is the best night of my life.

We met up at like 9 o clock at night and went to steak &

Shake. Then she came over to my place and we watched a movie. She then took some pictures with me and even smiled. It was amazing. Then she had on this cute hat and I pulled it off her head. I would say that if there was ever a time that I felt comfortable with someone that it was that night with her. After I pulled it off she made a confession to me. She told me that what I did was cute and that it would have been a good time for a first kiss. She knew I didn't have any experience in dealing with girls, so she was trying to help. I asked her if I could take her hat and try it again, but she said no, that the moment was gone.

Another week went by and then we went to a concert and watched a band. I got to dance with her a little, but this would be the last time that I ever saw her.

The Downfall

It was in late May that I also sold my trombone for $400.00. This was a professional trombone that was worth well over $2500.00 that I just gave away for $400.00 because I thought that that was the reason why no one liked me. Once again that feeling of being a band geek was stuck into my head. I had to change majors and become a business major because that was what the cool kids were doing.

After selling my trombone I became even more depressed. To me this showed me that music was a way of therapy for me. When I had my trombone, I was able to get away and escape into a make-believe world and play music. I couldn't get hurt there. Without that, there would be no escaping and there were many chances to get hurt.

It was during the spring semester of that year that I had also met another girl online and to this day we are still friends. Keck was reluctant to meet me in person but was okay talking online and texting. To this day we have only hung out three times in person. We text a lot and talk on Facebook periodically. She has also been a huge inspiration for trying to get through all of this.

One night my roommate was using my computer and decided that he was going to pretend like he was me and set up a hook up with Kecia. I immediately saw what he was doing and became worried that she was going to get mad at me. He was pretending to be me telling her that she should hook up with him. I immediately texted her and let her know what was going on and she gave him a number to some rejection hotline. When he found out he was furious with me and wanted to hurt me, but I didn't want her to be mad at me.

17 REACHING OUT

Finally, on June 17th of 2007 I had had enough and couldn't take it anymore. I was communicating with Kristen and Kecia and letting them know I was sad and wanted to kill myself. I had set up a place to hang myself on my balcony. I'm not sure if I would have gone through with it or not but I was very unstable at the time. Luckily the two of them got together and called someone and they got there just in time. I spent the next week trying to recover from that situation. I was in a behavioral unit at a local hospital.

Sometimes the things that are supposed to help us can hurt

us the worst.

During that week where I was supposed to be receiving help and encouragement I met a kid who was in there for drug abuse. During the week I told him my story and he said that it was crazy, and he was going to show me how to be cool and not get taken advantage of. So, he gave me his number and told me to call him when I got out of the hospital. I thought it was cool and maybe I was making a real friend.

When I got home I was recovering and trying to become happy again when I gave him a call. He said to meet him somewhere and that he was going to introduce me to a hot girl. So, I was like okay. Then when I got there. He said he needed to do some shopping but had forgotten his wallet at home and told me if I paid for his stuff he'd pay me back when we got to his place, so I did. Over $300 dollars' worth of stuff. New shoes, new clothes, and some other stuff.

Then he said he was going to run inside and grab some stuff and he'd be back and we'd go meet the girls. She has me park in an alley because he said he didn't want anyone to see we were there. He walked away. After a half hour, hour, and an hour and a half he wasn't back. After two hours, I finally gave up and left feeling used and abused again.

The next few weeks were spent trying to regroup and feeling depressed once again. My roommate was in and out of town, so the apartment was peaceful. He came back around the fourth of July. I just couldn't stand being hurt anymore and on the 3rd of July I had another suicide attempt.

This time I got in the car thinking I was going to run away and die somewhere. I ended up in Fun du lac, Wisconsin. When you are so misunderstood you have no one to go to. I thought that I was worthless, and no one wanted me here and thought possibly someone in Wisconsin or somewhere else might want me. If they didn't then I'd just kill myself there. So, after this trip I ended up in a hospital again. After this hospital stay I moved back in with my parents for like 3 weeks.

By the first of August I had met yet another guy who said he would befriend me and move in with me. He told me if I paid for an apartment he'd pay me, so I believed him and moved in. This guy never ended up paying me a dime and in fact ended up in jail. I got stuck paying for the entire apartment. I was only there two days and had to pay 3000 dollars just to get out of a lease. Once again, I was lost and confused and had no idea what to try or do next.

Switching Schools Yet Again.

By the time the middle of August rolled around, and it was time to go back to school I was still in a lot of emotional pain and didn't want to go back to Fort Wayne to go to school. So, I switched schools and went back to Indiana Wesleyan for the fall semester of 2007. I was going to live on campus this time and have roommates that were Christians. I thought that this was the cure. This was the solution for all my problems.

As the school year started things were calm and I was having fun. No one was being mean to me yet because they didn't really know me yet. During the early fall the group of guys from the unit I lived on would go play volleyball with a group of girls. These were normal college students doing normal things with other college students and I was being allowed to be a part of something like this for the first time in my life.

I felt like I was fitting in. I wasn't the coolest kid playing sand volleyball but at least I was fitting in. We would go grab pizza or something almost nightly after we played. It was great. However, as the semester went on I became more and more frustrated. It was hard for me. Yeah, I was able to play volleyball with these kids, but I still couldn't connect with them on a level to be able to be good friends with them. Again, it's the friendship/acquaintance ratio. I was an acquaintance to them, but I wanted them to be my best friends.

Schoolwork was hard. Not because I didn't know how to do it but because I was so focused on social interactions that I just couldn't even concentrate on schoolwork at all. By mid-October I was struggling socially again because it was getting cold out and the sand volleyball stuff wasn't going on anymore. I became more frustrated and depressed. After attempting to get some counseling several times through that university and being pushed away I didn't have anywhere to turn.

On October 30th of 2007 I ran again. This time I ran to Indianapolis. I ended up in a mall parking lot in Fishers,

Indiana which is just outside of Indianapolis and had a pair of scissors with me. I was sure that someway or somehow, I was going to end my life and get away from the world of pain. The funny thing is that sometimes people especially girls start paying more attention to you when you feel this way and want to kill yourself. They texted me and wanted to know where I was at. After about 5 hours of waiting in the mall parking lot I was finally able to tell someone where I was at and they came and got me.

Hospital #3....

This time when I got back I was forced by the university to go to a hospital. They obviously didn't want me anymore and just wanted to get rid of me. The school I was going to lied to my parents and told them that I had to drop my classes a week earlier than required by the university to receive a W instead of an F. They just didn't want to give me or my parents anytime to decide about it. Just because I was different I was a bother and they didn't want to deal with me. To this day I wonder if life at Indiana Wesleyan would have been different if they had known I had Asperger's syndrome.

Hospitals

Being put in the hospital for having Asperger's syndrome is such a waste of time and more depressing than being out of the hospital. I think it's funny that they think they're helping you by keeping you cooped up somewhere for a week. I wish they could come up with a better and more user-friendly way of helping people in need of help. After I got out of the hospital it was like we were back to the drawing board. Here we go again. Square one. I ended up taking the rest of the fall 07 semester off. I decided to go back to IPFW for the spring semester of 2008 and this time I would live on campus there.

Fall 08 at IPFW.

As January 2008 came along I was living with a random roommate I had never met before which was a horrible idea. I let myself get bullied again. Campus policy is that no significant other is supposed to be living there. Well this guy had his girlfriend living with him and it was just a 2-bedroom, 1 bathroom. I ended up being late to class in the morning quite a bit because of his girlfriend. She would just go shower whenever she wanted before she had to go to class and I was too afraid to say anything to them. I ended up doing bad in most of the classes from that semester.

People do things different when they're drunk than when they're not?

I learned a lesson this semester. I am not a drinker, so I didn't really know much about this at the time. But a girl who I'd met told me that sometimes when people are drunk they say and do things that they wouldn't do when they're sober. This made absolutely no sense to me. I still can't comprehend why someone would do or say something differently when drunk as opposed to being sober. It's like having two personalities. Well there was this girl that I danced with one time but at that time she was drinking. So, I started to try to dance with her again at another time because I thought she liked dancing the first time and she flipped out and got mad. She then explained the whole saying things when you're drunk vs. not drunk situation.

The rest of the semester at school was spent coping or should I say just dealing with what life had dealt to me. As you've noticed a common trend or theme throughout this book has been me trying to connect with women. It was in this time frame January 2008-June2008 that I would really start to try and make some discoveries about girls. In May of 08, a girl told me that she would go on a date with me if I did her homework. She had three final papers that had to be turned in and told me if I wrote them she would go out for coffee or drinks. So, I immediately started working on them. I ended up doing two of them because I was busy with my own stuff. It turns out that she never intended on hanging out with me. She was just wanting someone to write her paper for her. Little things here and there happened like this off and on for about a year from 2007-2008.

After surviving the summer without any social interaction again I was ready to go back to school. In August of 08 I was planning on attending IPFW to major in accounting. I was also offered a job and took it working with the YMCA. I ended up being afraid of going back to school. I couldn't do it because I knew the other students would hate me and make fun of me. So, I ended up dropping those classes and never going. The same thing happened in the spring semester of 2009. I signed up and then couldn't force myself to go. It's so painful to be made fun of and rejected all your life. I just couldn't do it anymore.

In the fall of 2008 I was so frustrated about my inability to connect with other people and especially girls that I goggled a phrase. I goggled "How do I get a girlfriend?" If you would ever Google that phrase there would be some interesting things that came up. I ended up spending about 5,000 dollars buying books or programs that I found on internet websites telling me how to get a girlfriend or how to attract girls. One of the more memorable programs that I got was a book containing text messages to send to women that would make them attracted to you. My favorite one that was in the book was the one that it said to use when asking a girl out. I was told to text a girl this. "Hey, I need to do some shopping. You should come along, and if you're nice, I'll even let you carry my bags for me. So, I tried some of these things out for a few months and found that nothing really worked. I was one of these people who thought that anything and anyone no matter who they were or where they were from would be out to help people in this world. I've had a few people who are helping me out tell me that the people I bought that stuff from was just wanting to make some money off me and had no intentions of helping me.

I can't comprehend why someone would just want to take money from people and not help them. Especially when it's something so serious. I hope that someday the world will start caring about people for who they are, and that people would put others before themselves and help them out.

In October of 2008 I met a guy at a club who wanted to help me out. Or so he said. I started talking with him and I told him my story and about how I wanted friends and wanted to learn how to talk to girls. He said he was a pro with girls and could teach me anything that I wanted. So, I started hanging out with this guy. As he told me he would be my friend and I could hang out with him and his group of friends if I paid him $500.00 a month. He told me he could teach me anything I wanted to know and help me get any girl I wanted to get. Before long we were hanging out and I was paying him. Then he started saying that I had to buy him and his friend's drinks whenever we hung out. So now I wasn't just paying him $500.00 a month but I was buying him and his group of friend's drinks.

After a few times of hanging out and him taking my money and really showing me nothing he told me that to get girls to like me I'd have to drink alcohol. To be cool and have other people like me he said that I needed to come over and do something called pregame. He made me buy a bunch of alcohol and bring it over and we started doing shots. He said that we needed to be drunk before we ever even went out so that we were cool. The more drunk we were the more girls would notice us. So, the first time I went over to his place I was told that we should do shots. We pre-gamed by doing ten shots of something. I didn't understand why I'd have to be drunk to be able to get a girl to like me. But he said that to be cool and attractive to girls I had to be wasted when I walked into a club.

I had never even drunk much at all before this. In fact, the only reason I even went to the club was to try and make friends or meet people. So, by the time I'd done ten shots and we went to the club I was already out of it and didn't feel well. Then while at the club I was told that if I gave him some money to give to girls that he'd get them to take pictures with me and dance with me. So, I did all of this. But by the end of the night the only one really getting pictures with girls and dancing with girls was him.

This went on for a period of two or three months. While I did meet some new people I never met anyone who offered to hang out with me for free or any girl who would take a picture or dance with me for free. To this day I still know and understand that to make friends I must pay people. I am not able to spend my financial aid money from school on things such as cost of living and food and that sort of thing. For the past 3 years all my financial aid refund has been used to pay people to be friends with me.

The frustrating thing is that a lot of adults and professionals in the field keep trying to tell me that I don't have to pay people to hang out with me or to be my friend. But they just don't understand it. I guess it's one of those things that you just can't comprehend or understand until you've lived with it and experienced it. I was having this conversation with a friend of mine named Charlie who is the same age as me and has Asperger's Syndrome. He shared that he shares some of the same frustrations as I do about making friends and trying to get girls to like us. He also felt that even professionals and older adults who are more understanding than our peer group still can't quite comprehend what it's like to have Asperger's Syndrome and live with it and its side effects daily.

After paying this guy for about three or four months and getting no results I finally had to quit paying him. In doing so I lost a friend. As a common person you might not think that someone charging me $500.00 a month to hang out with him on weekends was such a good friend but when you struggle with making friendships and fitting in with peers it was truly an enjoyable experience just to have someone to hang out with on a Friday and Saturday night. Unfortunately, as my financial aid money ran out my friend decided he couldn't hang out with me anymore.

There have been several other instances in my life in which I've been able to have a couple of friends. But to this day I've never had what I would call a good peer friendship with a guy without paying him to hang out with me. I've also not had any real dates with a girl unless I paid her to spend time with me or bought her a dress or something fancy that she wanted. The thing that I think is hard to comprehend for professionals and the average neurotypical person is how one can feel that he must pay people to hang out with him. The thing is, when that's the only way you've ever experienced a peer relationship with a peer that's just how you think it works. 500 professionals and 500 adults who are neurotypical could say to me "You shouldn't have to pay people to be your friend or to go on dates with you, but I won't be able to believe that until I see physical evidence of it.

I know that professionals and other adults who keep telling me I shouldn't have to pay anyone to hang out with me are just trying to help but the problem is that's all they keep saying repeatedly. But there's nothing to back that up with. There's not been a peer friendship develop without me paying this guy/girl a monthly or weekly fee to be my friend. There hasn't yet been a date with a woman who I didn't have to give 300 or 500 dollars for spending the evening with me. Or that I didn't have to buy something for to hang out with me. I can think of at least 25 different guys that I've paid to hang out with me and 12 girls that I've had to pay to spend time with me or go on a date with me.

It did seem like this guy really knew how to talk to girls and had a lot of success with them. He told me that I could hang out with him and his friends on weekends if I paid him a few hundred bucks a month. He said that he was doing me a huge favor because I was paying thousands of dollars for material that I bought from professionals on the internet and that a few hundred a month is cheaper than a few thousand. So, I took him up on it and tried it. It lasted for a few months. Basically, all I learned from him was that I had to be drunk and drink all the time to talk to girls. The friendship with him ended in late March or early April of 2009. I didn't have the money to keep paying people and I wasn't getting anywhere with girls or life. In March 2009, I was feeling really depressed and wanted to kill myself again. I stopped caring about everything. I didn't even go to work because I felt like no one liked me. There was a young teacher that worked at the school I was stationed at by the YMCA that I really liked a lot. I thought that a teacher might understand that I had Asperger's and possibly like me, so I sent her a card and flowers to tell her I liked her, and I think she got mad. It was around that day that I ended up visiting the hospital again do to suicidal thoughts. I never went back to the YMCA after that. I haven't worked since March of 2009.

Working

Some of the most recent statistics I have read say that only twenty percent of people living with Asperger's Syndrome have jobs. Of that twenty percent only, eight percent are in full time employment. It's easy to see why this is. For me as of right now I'm just scared to be around other guys. I know how guys are and how they can treat people and act. I was constantly beat up and abused at most of the jobs I've had throughout my life by guys. The thought of going to work somewhere makes me sick because it scares me that I'll get hurt. I'm also afraid of being taken advantage of. I've often signed over a paycheck to someone I work with because they've said, "You owe me your check just for me allowing you to work with me." Work is now known as a very dangerous and uncomfortable place for me. If I could work by myself then I would have no problem doing so.

The thing is in general people with Asperger's are often walking around at a huge disadvantage. We struggle with any little thing we try. I was just thinking today of how important social interaction is. It is the basis for anything we do in life. I no longer hear people saying, "I got a job because I knew how to do this." I hear them say "I got a job because I knew so and so who knew so and so." Success in life now has transferred over from what you know to who you know and when you have Asperger's there's not really much hope because you are horrible at social interaction.

Throughout the past two or three years of my life there

have been many things happen that have shaped who I am today, or should I say what I am. I've been in situations to where I saw a girl I thought was pretty and I wanted to talk to her. A few times these types of situations have ended with the girl saying "I'll give you my number if you give me $300 bucks. Or they might say I'll have drinks or coffee with you if you give me $500.00 bucks for my time. I have paid this quite a few times in fact I've used a lot of my financial aid money for this because I now know and realize I don't have any other choice and that this is the way it is for me.

In fact, just last night, I was at a dance club hoping to meet some new people. There were lots of pretty girls there. I tried asking about 10 of them to dance and they all turned me down. I got quite a few strange looks too. I was so frustrated. At the end of the night I finally got to dance with one girl. She came up to me and said she'd dance with me for $50.00. I gave her my last $50.00 I could get until 2 days later. This has happened so much to me that I know accept and expect to pay girls for any type of interaction with them. Even if it's just a simple hello, how are you? I would expect to offer her some money. I know that girls see me as not a person but as just a thing. I think they think that I don't have feelings, but I do so greatly have feelings. I guess I'm not expecting this to change anytime soon. I just know that if I'm ever going to date someone I would have to offer them 1000 or 2000 dollars per month.

Life with Asperger's.

While there are many different types of people in this world there are also people who have Autism/Asperger's Syndrome who are all uniquely different. As Stephen Shore says "Once you've met open person with Asperger's Syndrome, you've met just one person with Asperger's syndrome. I've found that in my time I've met people with AS who are content with it and okay with having it. These are the people that you won't even see trying to socialize with others. They're okay with it and just want to be alone. I however must think that this might be due to being rejected so much that they've just withdrawn from society which is a sad thing.

Then there are the people who are more like me. People who want and strive for that social interaction of a neurotypical person. The most frustrating thing is to be able to see the interactions of neurotypicals. It's like looking through a bullet proof glass window. You can see them all socializing and having a great time with each other, but you just can't figure out how to get there yourself. It's like I just don't have access to it. Either way happy with it or not it is what it is and it's something we all must deal with. There are times when I wish that instead of having Asperger's I had no legs or no hands. I feel like that might be better than having Asperger's because it's a visible thing and people tend to do better with that than something that is invisible. My advice for people with Asperger's is to seek out all the help and support you can get. It's also to be okay with who you are and appreciate life. This is something I still try to do and struggle with today. Lastly, educate people. Teach everyone you know about autism and Asperger's syndrome.

There is a lack of awareness in this world and this is something I'd like to see change.

Where am I today.

Today Travis is making another attempt at school. He's balancing a learning new social skill with learning numbers to be an accounting student. Life sometimes deals us many challenges and sometimes we deal yourself some of these challenges. I've spent a great deal of my life trying to figure out how to overcome the challenges by being someone different or being a book. No matter how much I could wish that I was someone else the harsh reality is that I'll always be Travis. I plan to finish my education and become a CPA at some point. I would also like to peruse another major in communications and travel around and speak to people about autism and Asperger's syndrome. If you're interested in contacting Travis, you may do so by emailing travisbreeding@gmail.com

A big thanks to everyone who read "Living without Knowing Who You Are" and learning a little about what it might be like to live with AS.

ABOUT THE AUTHOR

Travis Breeding lives in Huntington, Indiana. He graduated from Huntington North High School in 2004. Travis has a sister and resides with his family and a new niece that is part of his family. Travis was diagnosed with autism in October of 2007. He has a dual diagnosis of autism and schizophrenia. He shares his journey of how he learned to celebrate autism to help others live more meaningful lives. You find Travis on Facebook.